BEYOND BIRTH

A Mindful Guide To Early Parenting

By Sophie Burch

To Oliver, Milo, Reuben, Beau and of course PB.
I couldn't have created this without you.

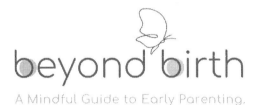

beyond birth

A Mindful Guide to Early Parenting.

Sophie Burch

Written by: Sophie Burch

This book is not intended as a substitute for medical advice. The reader should regularly consult a doctor in matters relating to their health or the health of their baby and particularly with respect to any symptoms that may require diagnosis or medical attention.

THE MAMMA COACH

YOU CAN DO THIS

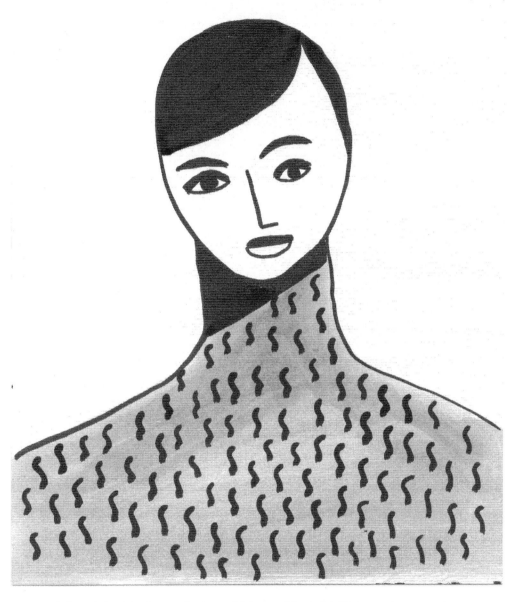

Artwork by kind permission of Margo Mcdaid: @margoinmargate

What people are saying about Beyond Birth...

'Attending the Beyond Birth Groups has been such a positive experience. It has helped me with those stressful, sleep deprived parenting moments and given me tools to respond instead of react. It's a journey in self development. I always leave feeling empowered and that it's ok to just be how I need to be that day.'

'The support of Sophie and the Beyond Birth Group was just what I needed after going through the bereavement of my mum the year before the birth of my baby and a difficult first 6 weeks. I left feeling energised and proud of what I had achieved in the past 6 weeks. My husband and I worked through the guide and our son is now 6 months old and everyday we both use what we have learnt not only with parenting but with our relationship and even in our work lives.

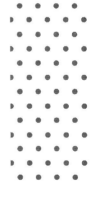

'Beyond Birth allowed all the emotions that I was scared to feel and process them without fear or guilt, as well as dealing with the day to day challenges parenting brings.'

What people are saying about Beyond Birth...

'Beyond Birth has been an invaluable part of our parenting journey and we are extremely grateful.'

'My wife and I are around 8 weeks away from our due date with our first baby, and we're using the lock down time to prepare for the birth and all that comes after. The Beyond Birth workbooks are forming a big part of that, so thank you for all that you've put into preparing those and all that you continue to do!'

'Motherhood has been a huge shock and also the biggest learning curve for personal growth too. Thank you for all your work - it makes a huge difference, I want you to know how much it is valued.'

'Beyond Birth is what's getting me through this if I'm honest.'

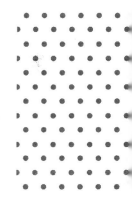

THE MAMMA COACH

What the experts are saying about Beyond Birth...

"The Beyond Birth Guide is a resource that I believe is an essential for any parent of a baby - regardless of whether this is their fifth baby, or their first.

As parents, we yearn for information and guidance as we enter parenthood, on how to navigate this life-changing transition in bringing new life into the world. We as parents are also 'born' again with each of our children, and this guide recognises, respects, and resources us in looking after our emotional, mental, and physical wellbeing during this process.

Importantly, there is focus not only on our relationships with our babies, but also our relationships with each other, and with ourselves. The guide is evidence-based and packed full of practical information and useful tools. It is invaluable not only because of the quality and research-basis of the information within the guide, but also because of the years of Sophie's experience and expertise that have been poured into the creation of this offering for parents.

The Beyond Birth Guide is an incredibly valuable resource in providing for and facilitating the emotional, psychological, and soulful nourishment we yearn for when parenting a baby."

Dr. Sophie Brock
drsophiebrock.com
The Good Enough Mother
AMIRCI President

What the experts are saying about Beyond Birth...

"This is a rich and warm guide for parents. Sophie's voice is one of kindness, she is so knowledgeable and there are so many lovely tips and tools in this guide. There is so much love poured into these pages. It's worth every penny. "
- Dr. Rebecca Moore
doctorrebeccamoore.com

"I wish that I had had The Beyond Birth guide after my first birth experience. Sophie offers tools for heart, body and mind, to make sure that we keep our own resilience at the heart of the story, knowing we cannot give endlessly in the way motherhood requires if we're not nourished internally in body and spirit.

What a beautiful support system for women at this incredibly vulnerable and powerful time of life. Thank you Sophie for providing the tools to grow and thrive through motherhood, and to be able to pass on this nourishment to our children through modelling it, being it."
- Anya Hayes
Author & Pilates teacher
Mothers' Wellness Toolkit
The Supermum Myth

"Sophie's guide offers much wisdom with an over-arching focus on self-compassion. This is so important for new parents, particularly in the early days of the transition, when it can feel so hard to look after ourselves alongside our baby. Sophie also includes helpful, normalising information about anxious, intrusive thoughts of harm about the baby which are so common, yet little talked about. Sophie offers nurturing, practical tips for coping and ways to develop self-awareness to help parents become more confident in their new role."
- Dr Caroline Boyd
Clinical Psychologist
Writer and Mother

THE MAMMA COACH

Contents

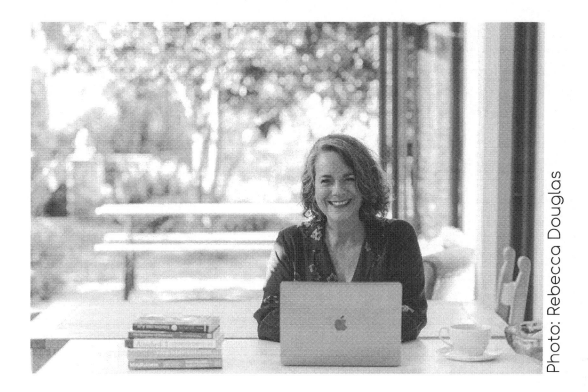

Photo: Rebecca Douglas

Foreword

Sophie Burch is mother to 4 boys (including twins), and is qualified in Hypno-CBT therapy including Mindfulness, IAIM Infant Massage and Aromatherapy (in addition to other complementary therapies). She is accredited by the CNHC and GHR.

Sophie's personal and professional experiences have inspired her to write this guide so that everyone can manage their mental wellbeing as they live through their baby chapter.

It's written for everyone, not just anyone struggling, and may serve as a preventative tool for mood disorders. Any information in this guide is derived from research and practice both personally and with clients.

THE MAMMA COACH

This is a mindful guide to help keep your mental wellbeing in balance, ease the transition and build resilience to help you cope with the worries and challenges of late pregnancy and early parenting.

There are 6 sections to explore, starting from the last few weeks of pregnancy and into parenthood for the first 12+ months.

I've designed this with both parents and caregivers in mind to develop or improve mental coping skills and maintain emotional balance during one of the most challenging, transformative times in human life.

It's evident now that we must educate and support ourselves more to manage the challenges of life as we know it.

Physical and Mental wellbeing are non-negotiable to maintain our health and rather than wait until we need specialist support, we owe it to ourselves and our children to take steps now, every day, to ensure a more resilient future for our families.

The lowdown:

A digital and virtual guide to connect with each other, expert professionals and other parents. Here are a few example of topics covered in this guide...

Nurture Self-care, self-love, healing, sleeping and resting.

Emotions Vulnerability, crying and basic infant neuroscience explained.

Connections Relationships and oxytocin.

Healing Recovery, forgiveness, gratitude, pain management, expectations, shame/guilt and fear.

Nourish Self, baby, mentally and using emotional language.

Transformation Movement, moving on, acceptance, new habits, facing fears, embracing vulnerability, acceptance and intuition.

THE MAMMA COACH

Welcome to this mindful guide for you; a pregnant or new parent. This guide has been designed to be the tonic you need to keep your mind in balance or help ease your worries as you find your way.

Together we'll work through the transition from pregnancy into parenthood.

Think of it as hand holding across a wobbly bridge into an unknown place, whereby you have some distant familiarity but could do with reassurance and help finding your feet. A bit like giving someone night vision glasses when trying to feel their way through the woods at night; learning skills to calm, soothe, and tune inwards for the answers. It's designed to help you find your identity as a parent (be it first or subsequent babies), and to connect with yourself, your baby and your loved ones.

I will be focusing on your psychological well-being, offering virtual support, ideas and questions to build resilience, cope with and accept the challenges, learn to trust in your instincts and intuition and feel confident when reaching out for help when required.

The early days of parenthood can be a roller-coaster of emotions leaving many people shocked at how they feel and wishing they'd been more prepared. By going through this guide, you are taking some big steps to doing just that.

Preparation, Preservation and Prevention.

Joyous and tough times in parenthood are very normal, and this guide is designed to help you find your balance on a mental and emotional level (which can and does lead to the physical too).

THE MAMMA COACH

This guide will give you skills that help you slow down, connect and ease the emotional intensity so you can enjoy and bank the first precious months instead of them going by like a blur and being forgotten.

It is not designed to be a mental health intervention. For anyone that may be struggling, if you feel that you need further help and are not coping please speak to someone close to you and use the resources included in the guide. If you find that you are experiencing the "baby blues" for longer than the first week, struggling to bond with your baby or more low or emotional than usual please speak to your healthcare provider.

Resources may differ from country to country, but wherever you are I would encourage you to also speak to your midwife, doctor, health visitor or general practitioner. The earlier you get help the better.

I would like to stress that whilst Mindfulness and Relaxation are great tools to use for coping, they are not recommended by the World Health Organisation and National Institute for Clinical Excellence as a remedy for those suffering from the symptoms of Post Traumatic Stress Disorder, whereby medical help may be required. There is a recommended self analysis form in the resources section that you can complete to see if you may need additional therapeutic or medical help. It's the same you would get at a GP appointment and will help any caregiver to assess how you are with regards to anxiety or depression.

How does it all work?

This guide uses a combination of mindfulness, relaxation, self-hypnosis, and other psychotherapeutic techniques as a self help toolkit over 6 sections. Some aspects you may be familiar with, and others not. You don't need to have heard or tried any of this before now to find it easy to use and simple to apply to life with your new baby.

Professionally created, the guide is designed for you to access whenever and wherever you choose from late pregnancy through the first year and beyond. It includes ideas sourced from evidence-based resources and personal experience as a therapist, coach and parent of 4.

You will have access to information sheets to download and links to go to online, mp3 tracks to save and listen to, and worksheets to get your thinking caps on and get to know yourself, your baby and your partner, better than ever before.

The guide is purely a guide. It's designed to help you to help yourself, but everyone is unique and what works for some may not for others, so please bear that in mind at all times. This is not meant as advice. It's meant to encourage you to think for yourself and recognise when you may need to reach out for help if or when you just can't manage.

THE MAMMA COACH

This is why I have created this guide for you

After 15 years working in the birth and baby world and having experienced mental health issues myself as a mother to 4 children and witnessing my partner struggle as well as hundreds of my clients, I believe we are missing a trick if we are not putting some preventative work into preparing for a baby. This is not just for anyone who is already struggling.

This is for EVERYONE who is preparing
for or already got a babe or two in their arms.

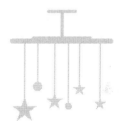

Here's what the UK
Mental Health Foundation says:

"Starting or growing a family is a milestone in many people's lives. It can also be a stressful time and many parents experience mental ill health. Mental ill health of parents can have a negative impact on the development of their children. But this is not always the case."

- During lockdown six in 10 parents said they had significant concerns about their mental health.
- Approximately 68% of women and 57% of men with mental health problems are parents.
- A perinatal mental health charity has said that it's seen a demand for support amongst men rise by 10%.
- It's estimated that one in five men experience anxiety after becoming a father and within the first year one in 10
- develops postnatal depression. The risk of depression continues after this time with a 68% increase in risk during the first five years of their child's life.

THE MAMMA COACH

Just breathe

When I talk about breathing in this guide, I'm referring to "conscious" breathing and not automatic breathing.

Automatic breathing is what we do to stay alive and we don't have to think about doing it, thank goodness!

Conscious breathing is when we focus on our breathing with an intent. It's usually from the diaphragm, in through the nose and out through the mouth, however, you may find that just thinking about your breath coming from your belly or ribcage rather than your upper chest will suffice.

When we breathe with focus, our parasympathetic nervous system (the "rest and digest" part of the brain) is triggered and releases hormones that help our body to calm, which leads to greater mental clarity. So, we are more capable of taking stock and considering our actions, rather than reacting (which is an effect of the stress response). Therefore, enabling us to relax a little and feel more balanced again. When combined with guided relaxation, this can have huge benefits to a stressed- out, exhausted, parent - or anyone in fact.

Now this is not always the instant fix though. Have you ever been in a situation when you were really stressed, and someone suggested you "relax" or "calm down"? You may have wanted to punch them. That's because you are in high alert mode; your mind has determined you need to go into defense mode and that means producing adrenaline and cortisol around your body, so you are ready to fight, flight, freeze or fawn.

THE MAMMA COACH

Everything will be ok. You've got this.

You won't be thinking much, other than being reactive and may not be capable of controlling your responses.

In that moment, the answer is within you, and what is helpful is either to walk away until you have had time to "defuse" or to do something to counter the fear/rage/anger/resentment/vitriol/hurt, or other another emotion you are experiencing. Perhaps screaming into a cushion, punching a pillow, crying, running fast up and down on the spot, or writing it all down until it's all out.

Anything, as long as it doesn't harm or frighten you or anyone else. This is okay. These emotions are normal, and we all have them.

Suppressing them can lead to a greater explosion or the emotion coming out in behaviours we feel are shameful or guilty about.

That old saying "it's better out than in" really is true.

What choosing to focus on the breath can do is help tremendously when we are able to think about what we can do to help ourselves. If we do this often enough, it becomes an "anchor" for us to help give us calm and clarity quicker and we are conditioned to it as a reaction to a stress trigger.

Not only does this enable us to cope with so much more in life, but it can help us as parents as we react to and around our children, enabling them to mirror us and learn to regulate their emotions and react in a more assured way as they grow.

Pause & reset

Relaxation has been used for centuries as a way for the mind and the body to de-stress.

Common ways to relax are massages, taking a bath or sitting down. However, in our modern day living, we are not particularly good at relaxing for so many reasons, so taking time to choose to relax each day can be hugely beneficial.

If we don't take time to relax, our minds and bodies go into overwhelm, overdrive and then we can become sick.

In this guide, there are MP3's to download that are designed to enable you to take time to be more mindful and relax.

It helps to have someone tell us how to relax, so there are guided relaxation tracks that make suggestions to you in order to help you give yourself permission to relax and let go of whatever it is you need to in those moments.

Based on mindfulness and applied relaxation techniques, they are easy and pleasurable to use.

Some people find they fall asleep when listening to the audio tracks, so please ensure you are not driving, operating machinery or on your own in charge of your baby - unless it's at a time when you are able to switch off anyway.

What is mindfulness?

Quite simply, this is a technique that's been used for centuries by Buddhist monks and is now becoming very popular worldwide because it's a simple, effective way to help deal with stress, anxiety, self-worth and worry.

It's about being aware of and in the present moment. The now. Observing your thoughts come and go as they pass by like watching the clouds in the sky. It's not about changing anything.

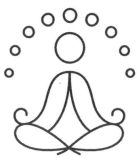

It's about accepting it and focusing on it until it passes by of its own accord.

Mindfulness can be useful to help focus within or around you and follow the sensations of your body, instead of fighting them. In parenting, it's an effective tool to help with moments of despair or loss of control and kids respond really well to it too, so it's something the whole family can practice together.

Have a look at this short video about Mindfulness as a SuperPower to gain a greater understanding and give you inspiration of how you can fit this into your daily life: https://www.youtube.com/watch?v=w6T02g5hnT4

THE MAMMA COACH

Look into my eyes...

Hypnosis is a
natural state of consciousness involving focused attention, reduced peripheral
awareness and an enhanced capacity to respond to suggestion (directive words
that suggest you do something).

It's like daydreaming.

You don't need to be able to relax completely to get into a "hypnotic state", but that can help.

It is NOT: Mind control and stage trickery... YOU CHOOSE.

Your belief and motivation to take part in this guide is all you need to succeed - and practice. Repetition ensures you can quickly become conditioned to behaving and thinking as you would like to. Just like learning something when you were at school, if you did it often enough, or were engaged enough, it usually imprinted on your memory. Self-hypnosis involves this, and a belief and motivation to succeed or make the changes necessary. Actively listening to the suggestions made to you by a hypnotherapist or on an mp3 and allowing yourself to follow the words and act on them enables.

ALL HYPNOSIS IS SELF HYPNOSIS

CBH (Cognitive Behavioral Hypnotherapy) combines Hypnosis and CBT and together they provide an effective solution therapy for anxiety, stress, low mood, insomnia and of course, childbirth, plus many more fears and phobias.

THE MAMMA COACH

Questions and journal sheets

This book has been designed so that you can put pen to paper and note down all that may crop up for you as you go through the guide.

Writing down your thoughts is an effective cognitive behavioral exercise that enables you to process with deeper reflection.

If you're not used to doing this, sadly many of us don't write much anymore, and the idea of "journaling" or answering questions may feel like too much effort or homework, then just add ideas to notes on your phone...

If you can push through this resistance, then you will reap the rewards. It doesn't all need to be tackled in one go.

Take one task at a time, or just one question at a time, or just bullet point what comes up for you.

Something very useful is about to happen for you.

THE MAMMA COACH

Something very useful is about to happen for you

Our thoughts can often lead to being a self-fulfilling prophecy if we use negative language like "I'm no good at anything." "This always happens to me." "I'll never succeed."

The language we use with others and ourselves has a profound effect on us at a deep, subconscious levels - quite simply, we can believe anything if we say it often enough because of the wiring in our brains - it's a form of conditioning. Or of creating habits, good or bad. The more often we repeat it, the more it will stick and become our belief.

Affirmations are statements that can help overcome negative thought patterns or a self-sabotaging mindset.

When you think about it, it's amazing that something so simple and free can have such an affect. Just like breathing, when we consciously choose to use words with intent, we can see lasting change.

Positive affirmations can work well to help us cement a new mindset about something we wish to achieve or believe about ourselves. However, firstly, they require a person to have a level of self-esteem and belief in themselves and the words they are using. When teamed up with visualisations, intent and positive thinking, affirmations can be life changing.

It does help to write your own affirmations, so that they are more meaningful and personal. To get you started I've created some that will help give you the confidence to create some of your own. Affirmations must be realistic, in the present tense ("I am), and said with feeling. It can help to say them in the mirror, but this can take a while to get used to.

Some people prefer to write them down and say them silently in their mind. This is okay if you really believe the words you are saying and the meaning behind them.

THE MAMMA COACH

Distance doesn't separate people. Silence does.

Talk to your partner or loved ones. Compare notes and celebrate this time. Make it special and document it as much as you can. Involve and ask for help from your family members and your friends. Or pop into the private Facebook group and ask questions - there will be people in there that will mostly likely be going through similar thoughts or feelings. I will be there for you too.

Do your best to reach out to your health visitors/care providers/doctors if you don't feel right or your thoughts and feelings are concerning you.

When to reach out:
We don't know the exact impact of the combination of someone's 'ghosts in the nursery': lack of sleep, pressures of work, finances and relationships and hormonal changes. Fluctuations are normal, to an extent. The "baby blues," for instance:
Up to 80% of new mothers experience mood swings, sadness, or anxiety soon after childbirth. But if you notice more serious symptoms, such as intrusive thoughts about hurting the baby or yourself, tell other people and seek support.

You can discuss symptoms with your doctor or go to a therapist for help. It's important to know that anyone, regardless of culture, age or history, is at greater risk for mental health challenges during the perinatal period.

This risk increases if you have a personal or family history of mental health problems; have experienced significant trauma; have a history of drug or alcohol problems; live in poverty; have major financial stressors; or if you don't have a good social support system.

Even with adequate support, postnatal depression or other mood disorders can occur, so it's even more important that we're talking and sharing about it so that we realize that PPD and other mood disorders are nothing to be ashamed of.

THE MAMMA COACH

A note on...

Birth trauma:

"One in 3 women find some aspect of their birth traumatic. This might be related to one or more events that happen before, during or after birth. It might be feeling out of control, fearful or powerless or fearing she or her baby was at risk. Partners, medical staff, friends, and family members may also have symptoms of trauma. The crucial element is that, at some point, the person felt that they or a loved one was unsafe." (Make Birth Better Cribsheet - Assessing for Birth Trauma)

Depression:

"The World Health Organisation predicts that by 2030 depression will be the leading cause of the disease burden globally"

WHO Executive Board, 'Global burden of mental disorders and the need for a comprehensive, coordinated response from health and social sectors at the country level'. (EB130/9 130th session 1 Dec 2011. Provisional agenda item 6.2)

Please see the PANDAS FOUNDATION or MAKE BIRTH BETTER websites for further information and signposting for support services.

THE MAMMA COACH

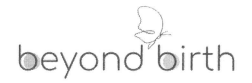

Nurture

HERE
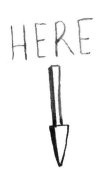

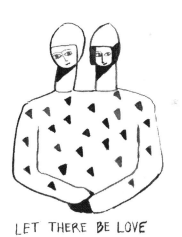

LET THERE BE LOVE

Definition:
To care for and
protect (someone or
something) while they
are growing

To help or encourage
the development of

To cherish

The action or process
of nurturing someone
or something

THE MAMMA COACH

"Mother-Nurture"

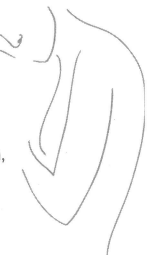

You may have come across the expression "Mother-Nurture", which implies raising and training our children, supporting and encouraging, educating and tending to them as the natural response in us drives us to do automatically.

This is also important to flip inwards and apply it to ourselves.

After the event of labouring and giving birth, our priority is focused on our baby and on recovery from birth.

Even if birth was "uneventful" with no intervention or medication, it will still have taken it's toll on both parents, usually starting in later pregnancy as the pressure for baby to come into our arms within given time-frames.

Never is there a greater time to be aware of our nurturing instincts.

We all have them, and we all have different ideas of what nurturing involves depending on our life experiences and how we were raised.

THE MAMMA COACH

What does 'nurturing mean to you?

Q: What does it mean to you to be nurtured?

Q: What thoughts, feelings and behaviours come to mind?

THE MAMMA COACH

Q: How can you nurture yourself? What do you need to do this?

Q: How can you nurture your baby?

Q: How can you nurture your partner/loved ones?

Within the subject of nurture I have included:

- Sleep/rest
- Self-care
- Self-love
- Healing
- Support.

THE MAMMA COACH

"Emotional
regulation flows
naturally
from being in the
presence of
someone we trust"

— Bonnie Badenoch

Shhhh (Zzzzzzzz.....)

Will you get any?

Most people know that a new baby brings interrupted sleep, but what many people don't quite grasp is just how this affects us on every level.

Society has conditioned us to pray for "a good sleeper", but what we don't perhaps accept is that all babies need short sleep/awake cycles.

So the kindest thing to do is to go with the flow, rather than force longer sleep times or follow sleep training advice for at least the first 6 months. The amount a new baby sleeps depends on so many factors and we just can't know from day to night to day what that will be. This is why counting how much sleep we get and saying things like "I only got two hours", is going to set us up for feeling like we are failing.

Changing our attitude and language to sleep and sharing the care can be big steps towards feeling better about it and being more accepting of how it is for the time being.

Thinking of the quality of the sleep you have rather than the quantity.

Catching deep restful times while listening to an MP3 or Yoga Nidra track for 20 - 30 minutes can be the equivalent of several hours of fitful sleep.

I'm tired. That is all.

Being tired, leads us to feel vulnerable, irritable, and often like we are the only one who is tired. We begin to measure sleep; longing for a "good" sleep and comparing it with our partner or others with new babies.

Lack of sleep is tortuous and there's no getting away from that feeling when we absorb with it and allow it to drag us under.

Fight it and we generally feel worse.

Judgement and comparison can lead us down a very dark internal path of envy, jealousy and possible rage.

We may say things we don't mean and feel agitated by the smallest of niggles. This can make us feel like we are alone, failing and at worst, losing our minds.

A distant memory of our previous perky, sleep-fuelled selves. It can tip us into blaming ourselves and others; our self-critic goes into overdrive and dare anyone try and give us advice, or, we get into a pickle about all the advice out there and end up feeling confused, worthless, and "a bad parent" before our parenting chapter has even begun.

We shut down and lose the ability to reach out for fear of baby being taken away or being judged as a bad parent - and tiredness can blow these thoughts out of proportion very quickly and may lead to mental illness if it's not remedied.

THE MAMMA COACH

Invest in rest

We all need different amounts of sleep, but if you are feeling sick with tiredness and can't think straight then caffeine may keep you going briefly, but it can't replace quality sleep.

This is not meant to be a section on sleep advice and I'm by no means an expert, but there are a few common sense ideas that may help.

How you do it is unique to you, but remember that being as flexible as you can and adapting where necessary will ease the ups and downs.

So how can we cope?

- Be kind and compassionate. To yourself, your baby and your partner - this will pass. You will get sleep again. Use daily affirmations and mantras to help keep you on a more positive track: "This will pass", "I am enough", "I take time to take care of myself and rest when I can".
- Tap into the hormones that help you sleep. Create a nest and keep the chores and visitors to a minimum until you feel you can get into a routine which could be many months away. Cuddles, feeding, low lighting, skin to skin, music (nature sounds can be very soothing), quiet voices, kind words, baths and massage can all set the mood.
- Attachment helps baby and you feel more aligned together and secure, but it's also ok to have time apart, when baby is asleep if there is someone there to help.

THE MAMMA COACH

- Use meditation mp3's or yoga nidra tracks to rest deeply when you can. Use the free audios provided as often as you can.
- Share the sleeps and the feeds with your partner, family member, friend or professional.
- Educate yourself to understand sleep and baby sleep patterns.
- Try not to force the sleep times. When baby is older and more naturally going into a routine by themselves, sleep routines should happen.
- Keep baby with you, but safe in a cot/crib if you're going to sleep unless you really can't sleep with baby near you, then take it in turns with your partner to sleep in another room in chunks of four hours.
- Use earplugs when you are not on baby duty.
- Remember to reassess often. Circumstances change frequently with a young baby and it's okay to change your mind if you are becoming stressed and overtired. It's not a sign of weakness, it's a strength in versatility.
- If you feel resentful of your partner, or like you are failing somehow, try to see where that is coming from. How realistic is it? How are those thoughts and feelings working out for you right now?

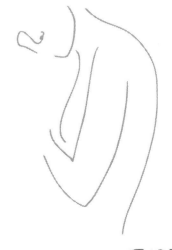

THE MAMMA COACH

Self-care is giving the world the best of you instead of what's left of you.

You've probably seen and heard this phrase bandied about everywhere. Just like Mindfulness, society is cottoning on to the fact that we are a stressed bunch who spend long hours working with not much to off-set the accumulation of pressure.

Both Mindfulness practice and self-care are being proven to help redress the balance as we search for quick fixes to slow us down, pause, let off steam and understand why our busy minds and stiff bodies that are sat at desks or on sofa's need some solace. Up to now, you may have had time to go to the gym or a yoga class.

Play about with the latest meditation apps or enjoying long weekend walks with family or friends after a fun night out.

You may have bought a journal or been given one, but don't really stick to writing in it. Isn't that what teenage girls do? Write a diary?

Sometimes the simple things we do for ourselves that we take for granted are the things we miss the most when we stop doing them, and we realise how good they actually were for us.

> You deserve to flourish and the only person
> that can really do something about it is you."
> – Suzy Reading, 'The Self-Care Revolution'

Don't feel guilty doing what is best for you.

Alongside joy, connection and love, a baby brings feelings of disconnection with our pre-baby selves.

In addition to the tiredness, we busy ourselves putting the baby first in everything we think and do.

The thing to note, is that if we don't reconnect with ourselves in a way that brings us home and helps us feel content on an emotional, mental and physical level, we will soon burn out, feel resentful, have regrets and lose our self-belief and self-awareness.

Self-care is not selfish, it's necessary.

It's simply a way to top up our energy banks every day so that we can take care of our babies and our loved ones. It's the ultimate act of nurture and nourishment.

Self-care is about the little things that top you up in the day and night. It could be a big treat, like having a haircut, a massage or a manicure, but mostly, it's the things we have easy access to, like a walk in nature, cuddles on the sofa, your favourite food, lighting a scented candle, or listening to music that lifts your mood or relaxes you.

Taking time to take care of yourself in this way does so much for our feelings of self-worth and self-awareness. It helps us to take a pause and focus on our needs for a while.

Even a few minutes spent savoring something delicious or taking a few slow, deep breaths can adjust the balance and top up our energy banks. Leaving us feeling subtly stronger, less wallowing and tuned-in much more to our intuition.

Self-care is also about the language we use to ourselves.

Being aware of that harsh inner critic and instead, using kinder words, talking to ourselves as we would do a friend.

To give you an idea, self-care can be broken down into sections to help divide up the tasks you can do:

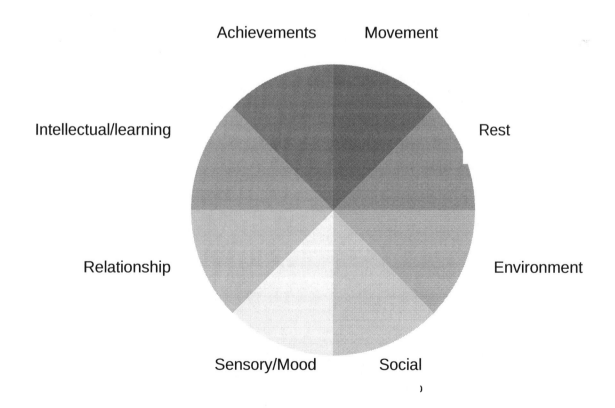

THE MAMMA COACH

Q: What would you include as your self-care essentials? Make a list and put a copy in places you can see several times a day to remind yourself to make micro-moments of time for yourself.

Q: What can you do at least once a week that will feel like a treat?

THE MAMMA COACH

Q: What words or phrases can you use that feel like acts of self-care just by saying them to yourself?

It helps to add things to a calendar and schedule in time for you. Could you do this? If not, what would be a good way to establish small acts of self-care into your daily routines? Don't worry about feasibility, brainstorming along the way is helpful. As I said before, be adaptable and flexible in your approach and fresh ideas will come.

THE MAMMA COACH

Life is too short to spend it battling with yourself.

It all starts with you and comes back to you.

I hear you.

Easier said than done? Yes, it's a tough one.

Why? Because the majority of us are riddled with self-doubt and a very active inner critic.

Becoming a parent is a time when the attention is on the baby, and in some ways it's required for us to become more "selfless" than ever before, however, in order to be truly capable of caring for this new life we've brought into our arms, we must first draw our attention inwards and reflect on how we can love and care for ourselves so that we are most able to be loving, kind and compassionate for others.

If we don't know how it feels to suffer, how can we be compassionate to others?

"If you can love yourself, you will be able to love others and others will love you right back."
- Sophie Burch, The Mamma Coach

The word compassion means "to suffer with". Therefore, knowing how to comfort and care for yourself, will give you a safe place to heal, being flexible and understanding when challenges arise in yourself or others you place your trust in.

Who said we were supposed to be perfect anyway?

Being a good parent is hugely different from being a perfect parent.

Being self-critical and judging yourself on every mistake, big or small, often results in feeling like a failure, frustrated and not honoring your humanness. Who wants to bring up a child demonstrating that is the best way to be? No. We want the best for our children. To teach and protect them.

The most important things we can teach them are not academic; they are to have love and compassion for themselves and others.

Kristin Neff says: "Self-compassionate people recognise that being imperfect, failing, and experiencing life difficulties is inevitable, so they tend to be gentle with themselves when confronted with painful experiences rather than get angry when life falls short of set ideals." (Self-Compassion.org)

THE MAMMA COACH

"You can only do your best"

Have you heard this before? Most likely you have.

How did it make you feel?

Did you welcome it and accept that as fact, or did you still resist it and strive to do better because that's in your nature?

Do you feel like "Just doing your best" is as good as saying you're not doing enough? Or are you happy to sit in the "Good enough" camp and be done with it?

Being good enough has different meaning for everyone and invariably it goes back to how we were raised by our parents, the education system we were in and then into the work we did and do now.

The world of work is rife with comparison and slogans everywhere telling us to be and do "Our Best".

We have to make everyone proud.
We have to be number one.
We have to get it right.
Be our most productive and have it all.

When we turn to parenting, naturally, we want to apply the same logic, ruleset and life habits to this and when we can't control it, we feel like we are failing. Miserably. Out of control. A sign of mental wellness is accepting that no-one is perfect.

Self-compassion is simply giving the same kindness to ourselves that we would give to others.

This is where self-compassion comes in.

By taking a balanced approach to our negative emotions, we are able to observe them instead of burying them or blowing them out of proportion.

We can't ignore our pain and mistakes and feel compassion at the same time, so by being mindful we are able to 'diffuse' before we absorb into those negative emotions and thoughts.

We are all human and we are all unique and come with our own set of nuances. Babies included.

Your baby will love you no matter what and will mirror your behaviours, setting them in stone for life.

We live in an imperfect world, so accepting that you are flawed is a valuable life skill and lesson learnt.

Now is the time to learn to love and be compassionate to yourself, self-soothing and being self-sufficient; and your child will follow suit.

Tips and Ideas to nurture your self-love and self-compassion

- Become mindful in your actions.
- Act on what you need rather than what you want.
- Practice good self-care. People high on self-love nourish themselves daily through healthy activities, like nutrition, exercise, proper sleep, intimacy and healthy social interactions.
- Set boundaries. Say no to work, love, or activities that deplete or harm you physically, emotionally and spiritually.
- Protect yourself. Bring the right people into your life.
- Forgive yourself. We can be so hard on ourselves. Remember, there are no failures, if you have learned and grown from your mistakes; there are only lessons learned.
- Live intentionally.

Become aware of your inner voice. Be aware how you treat yourself.

We all talk to ourselves in our minds, but we are not always fully conscious of that voice. Become conscious of your inner voice. Pay attention to what it's saying.

Sometimes we are so used to hearing it, we find it hard to hear it or notice we have one at all.

What do you say when you do something well, and what do you say when you fail?

Here are a few examples of situations in which you can keep awareness of your inner voice:

When you wake up and look in the mirror
When somebody is mean to you
When you are mean to someone
When you act on your anger
When you see a person in need but you keep walking without helping them
When you put on weight
When you make a mistake
When you eat unhealthy food
When you lie to somebody
When you make someone cry
When you feel lazy
When you don't do what you set out to do
When you rest

Take control of your inner voice

The things you hear in your head now have been there all your life.

You've been feeding yourself these messages for years, and the more we hear something, the more we believe in it. Which means that all the negative or positive things you say to yourself have become your strongly held beliefs.

This may feel pretty permanent, but these beliefs can be changed with some motivation and repetition. If you can tune in and listen to your inner voice, next time you catch yourself saying something unkind, pause, and say

"that's unkind, delete, delete"

It's a strange little trick, but it actually sends a message to your subconscious mind to ignore what you just thought. Crazy!

After noting it and deleting, say something new, this time a supportive, loving and caring message. And just keep doing it.

For example: "That's ok, I'll remember it next time."

At first, it may feel like a lie and your critical mind will resist and dismiss it. You may not believe in it at all and that resistance is normal and ok.

Keep doing it and over time, you'll become neutral to the message and finally you will believe it.

Treat yourself like a child

Having your own child is a time when your childhood memories and experiences often come flooding back.

So never was there a more important and poignant time to process some of this and get to grips with your inner child.

After years of having an inner critic and sometimes inner cheerleader, people often wonder how they should talk to themselves differently. Being so harsh on ourselves for so long means we don't know what that new voice sounds like. So to help you change the tone of your inner voice, imagine yourself as a child. Some people call it your inner child.

Tuning into your inner child allows you to look at yourself without the same judgement.

See yourself as a little, vulnerable innocent child, that simply wants to be loved. Perhaps you can remember yourself as this child?

We all have an inner child within us, just as we have an inner wise one too. There are needs that may not have been met when we were very young – and we carry those needs into our adult lives.

We might suppress them, push them into subconscious and not even realise they are there, but there are.

Now is the time to tune into those and give yourself what you needed then.

You carry so much love in your heart. Give some to yourself.

Love yourself emotionally and physically.

To love ourselves in parenting is a powerful gift to give to yourself and your baby. They will mirror you and what you feel will radiate to them and your loved ones.

What do you do when you love someone?

Think of your parents, siblings, a lover or a best friend.

Do you compliment them?
Do you buy them gifts?
Do you spend quality time together?

Love is a feeling and an act. So do something loving for yourself with intent - feel into it as you would do for anyone and you will reap the rewards. We all have a love-language, what's yours? It may be different to your partners (if you have one), so working this out now can really help in the long term.

From now on, give yourself permission to do things you enjoy. Even with a young baby in tow, you can manage to squeeze some in.

THE MAMMA COACH

How to start 'practicing' self-love and self-care

- Write in a journal.
- Listen to a soothing meditation/a podcast you enjoy.
- Do something creative (draw, paint, make, photograph)
- Talk to yourself as you would do a beloved friend. Use kind language to yourself and write down 3 things you like about yourself.
- Cook something you desire.
- Drink a smoothie or a hot chocolate or just savor your next cuppa.
- Read your favourite book.
- Watch or listen to comedy.
- Buy yourself something to wear.
- Book a massage.
- Go to a yoga or pilates class or take 20 minutes to cycle around the block or through a nearby park.
- Dance and go perfectly crazy in your house.
- Listen to your favourite music.
- Walk in nature or just around the neighbourhood will be fine - do it mindfully and notice what you see that you've never seen before.
- Do nothing. Yep – just sit, or lie down and do absolutely nothing. It's harder than you think! The more you practice acts of self-love, the stronger message you send to yourself:

"You deserve it" and "You are enough".

Write your own list and set an intention to do at least 2 things from your list each week.

Support

The reason I've included this under the nurture section is that support is an act of nurturing yourself or of others. If a parent doesn't feel supported on every level, the house of cards can soon come crashing down.

Getting support is something we as a society are not particularly good at these days. Years ago, it was the village that raised the child, but now, with more of us living in "nucleus family" situations, we are used to fending for ourselves and some feel it's a sign of weakness to ask for support, may be ill equipped to find the confidence to do so or in denial we need any until it's too late.

This is proven to pile on the pressure and we are seeing relationships failing and mental ill health on the rise. Families living further apart and couples working longer hours, can mean families inadvertently cutting themselves off from any help at a time when they need it the most at arguably the biggest transformational time in their lives.

The good news is, if you know where to look, there is a great deal of virtual support out there, like this guide, if you're into DIY support. The not-so great news is that new parents are often on their own in the community and have to work hard to reach out and research where the local support, baby-groups and new parent friends are.

Not everyone has the funds to join an NCT group or equivalent and unless you have a history of mental illness and so on. The system is not set up to reach out and offer much at all. It does depend on where you live, as some areas have more on offer than others, but it varies enormously, and what's on offer is not to everyone's taste.

A main downside to asking for support is that most of it comes with conditions. Some clearly visible and some unsaid. Not everyone has your views and may offer advice that goes against your values or doesn't sit well with your intuition. However, if we cut ourselves off because we don't want to face these people/places/offerings, we may find ourselves alone and isolated. Which can lead to mental ill-health if you're not careful.

THE MAMMA COACH

Support can be emotional, mental or practical, so it helps to list your ideas under these headings. Let's begin by asking a few questions:

Q: How do you feel about support?

Q: What support do you currently have?

Q: What support would you like?

Q: How are you going to ensure you have what you need and where are you going to get it?

Q: How are you going to manage without any?

Q: How are you going to manage with support you feel you don't want/need?

THE MAMMA COACH

The way you
speak to yourself
matters.

Affirmations

I take care of my needs

I take time for my self-care

I can support myself and ask for help when I need to

I am aware of my limits

I create boundaries where needed

I love myself

Self-care is not selfish care

I nurture myself as I nurture my baby

I am aware of what I need today & take steps to ensure I am ok

I am enough

I love my body, it has created and performed miracles

I trust in my body

I take care of my mind as I take care of my body

I nurture myself as I would nurture all my loved ones

Today I go at my own pace

Sometimes it's ok to do nothing

I take time to listen to my inner voice

I trust my intuition

I follow my instincts

Despite how tired I feel, I nurture myself in any way I can

Small steps, every day

Your Affirmations

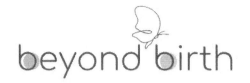
Emotions

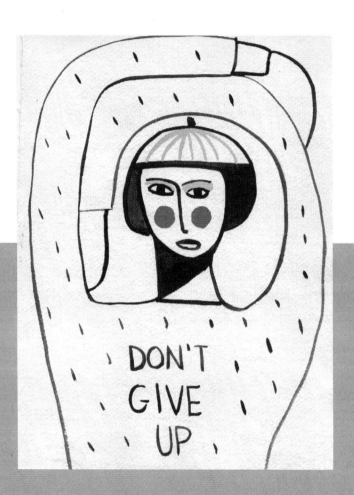

"Our body instinctively knows what it needs to do to process an emotion. We were born knowing how to externalise our feelings, and then we were taught to suppress them. It's time to start honoring our emotional needs again."

- Chantelle Sawden

Ups and downs

Bringing a baby into your life can be like being on an emotional rollercoaster. It ideally starts with a fierce, unparalleled love, deep feelings of warmth, connection, a desire and need for safety, security and having needs met. However, this is not always the case.

How we feel when we meet our baby for the first time is unique to everyone.

What a mother feels, is not the same as what the father or partner feels. Same goes for siblings, grandparents, and anyone caring for your baby. The emotion we feel can't be measured, compared or described in words. Those moments are so precious and we want to remember them, but often, depending on circumstances, those moments flit by and disappear into the haziness of our tired minds.

Depending on how pregnancy, labour and birth went and circumstances afterwards and other factors such as how we were parented, past trauma etc., the emotional bond we feel with our baby may be instant or grow over time.

Much of it depends on hormones and closeness, which we will cover in the "Connection" section of this guide. Whatever happens, having a baby stirs up strong, deep emotions in everyone and it's how we manage what crops up for us that matters.

Uncertainty, risk and emotional exposure

Vulnerability: the quality or state of being exposed to the possibility of being attacked or harmed, either physically or emotionally.
(source: Google dictionary)

Giving birth is a huge mental, emotional and physical experience that lays us bare. We have to give in to our vulnerability in order to give birth however we choose to or however it happens.

Birth is also the moment of physical separation of baby, from the mother and a moment of profound connection for a partner when baby lands in their arms. Becoming a parent lays us bare to our most vulnerable state.

Bringing a helpless baby into our arms, challenges us to step up and be the responsible protector, often without much previous experience if it's the first baby, or if it's a subsequent baby, then there are additional complex layers too.

Both parents (if there are two parents involved), will feel this vulnerability in differing ways but it doesn't mean one is more or less than the other.

Being vulnerable triggers our brain to release the stress hormones cortisol and adrenaline so we are alert and ready to react; useful in rare situations of extreme danger, but mostly redundant in reality. Therefore, being aware of this and managing it with techniques to comfort and reassure our vulnerability is going to serve new parents well as they navigate the minefield of early parenting.

Do you think it's ok to be vulnerable?

Q: What does vulnerability feel like to you?

Q: What steps can you take to allow yourself to be vulnerable and be ok with it?

THE MAMMA COACH

"When we feel shame, we have a terrifying fear of rejection. When we feel worthy, we trust in the opposite of rejection, we have a sense of acceptance and belonging. Vulnerability is the state we exist in when we can hold onto both fear of rejection AND a sense of self worth"

— Brené Brown

Crying is how your heart speaks

The main emotional response we are talking about here is crying.

Be prepared for tears.

Happy tears and tears of anguish and of sadness. Tears from you and many, many tears from your baby.

We are conditioned to respond to crying, which is one of the reasons a baby cries; so we do something about it. It makes us react.

Now that can feel unbearable at times, especially in the early months when crying peaks and we are not accustomed to it yet. But mostly, once we are conditioned to our babies crying, we take it to mean something.

Babies have different sounding cries for what they need at the time and although most parents would say they don't hear the differences or consciously understand what that is at first, subconsciously/intuitively, they automatically respond in the way their baby needs.

Some are more vocal than others, but this does not translate to them being a "difficult" baby, a label which society is often happy to pin onto any baby that cries, anywhere, anytime.

THE MAMMA COACH

Baby emotion

A baby cries because they are hungry, tired, need changing, are in pain, crave a cuddle or need entertaining. We cry because we are tired, angry, in pain or need a release. When we cry it's mostly emotive. When a baby cries, it's mostly communicative.

This is the difference, but as adults, we are conditioned to interpret crying as deeply emotional and not something to tolerate easily, which is why when our baby cries, it's hard for us to cope on an emotional and mental level. It can send us into "headless chicken" mode or into "high alert" to deal with it (and make it stop), which is why we are sensitive to what others think of us at that moment too.

In that mode, cortisols and adrenaline are released to ensure we react, which is why it's hard to calmly deal with a crying baby if they have been doing so for a while.

Mentally, if a parent is living with a baby who cries a great deal, it can have the same effects on them as stress. Another reason to get support and share the care if you can.

Not wanting to be alarmist, but lots of research has gone into our early brain development and studies have shown that if babies are left to cry for long periods, we may be doing a great deal of damage to their brain pathways; their ongoing distress can result in a reaction of hormones that are toxic to their brain and nervous system, leading to despair and dissociation and brain cell death in the emotional brain.

Quite simply, they become so fearful, they shut down. So to us, it may look like a baby being left to "cry it out" is learning to self-soothe after a while because they go quiet and fall asleep, but what could be happening is far more distressing and can have life-long emotional damaging effects possibly leading to mental health issues and heightened reactions to stress and other life challenges.

Babies need help with emotional regulation. They need to be comforted when they cry and shown that it's safe to express their needs, rather than shut down and rejected.

Naturally, this will lead to more problematic behaviors as they grow older. It's not building a rod for your back. It's showing love, kindness, compassion and offering safety and freedom to be heard.

Sometimes in life we just need a hug, no word, no advice, just a hug to make you feel you matter. Being held and being heard is a basic human need and right. It can promote deep emotional healing and help us to grow in trust, empathy and compassion for others. Now, I'm sure that's what you want for your baby?

If not, what are your reasons?

Q: What one thing would you gift a new parent, that would help them in the first year

A: I would gift a mum-buddy. A reassuring wise woman who could be there with reassuring words, cuddles for her and baby and who could do practical things too"

— Julianne Boutaleb, Consultant Perinatal Psychologist, Parenthood In Mind

What are your thoughts on crying?

How does crying affect you?

THE MAMMA COACH

What do you think and do when you see someone else cry?

What are the signs of stress on the body?

What can you do to manage these times?

What thoughts do you have right now?

How realistic are they?
Can you rationalise them?
Can you talk to yourself as you would do a friend?

Top tips to cope with a crying baby

If you have addressed all their needs and baby is still crying, and you don't think they are in pain, then try the following:

- Understand that it's not personal, it's a process. Your baby needs to cry right now and all you can do is comfort them. Reassure them with kind words and gentle, loving touch.

- Being on alert yourself, your mind is switched into safety mode: do what you can to reassure yourself that this is not a situation to fight, flight or freeze; your baby needs you to be rational and calm and you can do this by affirming to yourself that you are safe. Place your hand over your heart and say "I am safe", "I am held", "I am ok", "This will pass"

- Take 3 deep breaths in through your nose and out of your mouth. Relax your upper body, softening your shoulders and jaw: breathing in this way helps to trigger inner calm and soothe us. If you are holding baby, ensure you are supported and baby will notice as you breathe and still yourself. The longer you can do this the more likely your baby will mirror you.

- Ground yourself by imagining your feet are growing roots into the ground, sturdy and strong. Rock, sway and gently create a rhythmic voice and hypnotic movement to help soothe you both.

- Change scenery; go for a walk, pop baby in a sling and pace around, or lie down with baby and try to relax together.

- Know your limits. Recognise your internal warning signs. If it's getting too much, call a friend/family member and talk about how you're feeling.

- Remember that time is on your side: this will pass.

- You don't need to be able to meet your babies needs all the time - there's no such thing as the perfect parent. Experts estimate that meeting your infant's needs at least <u>one third of the time</u> is enough to support healthy bonding and secure attachment. Don't worry about getting it exactly right all of the time. Instead, try to relax and enjoy the times when your baby isn't crying.

- Having skin to skin can help produce the oxytocin and endorphins you both need to reconnect and calm.

- Find a Mantra for the moment: "I am enough. I love my baby and my baby loves me. It's okay to find this hard. I am coping as best as I can"

Attachment and the baby brain

I'm no expert in parent and baby neuroscience, but over the years I've read, researched, experienced and seen the effects of love, attachment and brain development for both baby and parent. It is the nucleus of the family cell.

In her book "Gentle Birth, Gentle Parenting", Sarah Buckley, MD., talks about the physiological stability between a parent and baby; the homeostasis that exists, calling it Mutual Regulation.

"Mutual regulation involves you and your baby exchanging information and influencing each other's body processes for on-going well-being and optimal development."

If we are unloved as infants, we are unregulated and unwired. Neglect can be as harmful as abuse and trauma to a baby, therefore leaving big "unwired" gaps in their brain development, especially around the emotional/limbic brain. If this happened to us as children, as parents, we may have issues to work through around attachment, how we are social, how we self-regulate our emotions and we may possibly have a predisposition to anxiety, depression and a lack of empathy to others; which can affect how we are with our own babies. All evidence suggests that early loving and attachment is even more important to our brains than early learning for our cognitive development - a healthy, well-functioning brain.

THE MAMMA COACH

This is not implying that if you ever leave a baby to cry for short periods, it's going to be damaging for life, no. In fact, brief times of crying on their own can teach older babies that negativity can be endured and overcome. Crying can help to heal and repair past traumas, so having our emotional response of crying instantly shushed, may not always be a good thing.

It's more important that a baby knows we are there and will comfort them, even if it takes a little while. Just the same with us, a good cry on our own can actually make us feel better by release. It's an impossible task to fulfill all babies needs and calm all stresses, but being available can mean everything. Telling someone to shush when they are crying can be seen as silencing them, rather than being present and listening.

Saying, "I'm here, it's OK, tell me all about it" can go a long way to holding space for someone to be open, express how they feel and let go of their emotion.

If we can do this for our babies and children, they are more likely to do this with their loved ones too. Same with our partners. Holding space for them to free their emotions, especially in the early months of parenting can be just what the doctor ordered, instead of rushing in trying to fix it with suggestions and judgements. This is called an empathetic response.

This short video demonstrates how important early attachment is for us and why: https://www.youtube.com/watch?v=WjOowWxOXCg

Life skill

Dealing with strong emotional responses is something that every parent faces on a daily basis. Having conscious ways to help cope is a valuable life skill that can be used throughout parenting and life. Instead of being reactive, which can lead to shame, guilt and inner child-like behaviors, we can learn to respond in ways that allow us the grace to feel more measured in our reactions and most importantly safe and in control.

Here are a few suggestions for you. Firstly, let it R.A.I.N:

RECOGNISE - the thoughts and feelings that are causing a stir.

ALLOW - let whatever is there be there, without changing it or fighting it. This can be hard as the resistance is strong. Deepen your attention on it.

INVESTIGATE - Observe it and see what's what and why. Get your detective hat on. Notice the feelings and how the thoughts affect how you feel. Ask yourself, "what do I most need right now"? Trust the answers you get.

NURTURE - Be kind to yourself. Use self-compassion to allow yourself to feel held and safe. Feeling heard and softening into it all, knowing you are experiencing a human reaction to something you most likely have very little control over.

THE MAMMA COACH

Visualisation exercise - childhood reflection

You can do it just by reading the text below to each other or having a quick read through and going over the idea your own way. Having a journal to hand to write down what crops up for you might be useful.

Before you begin:

This can potentially be triggering if there has been childhood distress or trauma, so I'd suggest talking to a professional therapist if you can. Please see resources for some recommended services or research a local therapist who is trained in working with the perinatal period.

If you are able to and have memories of your childhood that you feel you can reflect on, then find a safe space to sit and get comfy. Then, take a moment to reflect back to your childhood, and write down some of the emotional memories that come up for you. When you felt happy, sad, angry, excited, confused, hurt, joyful and so on.

Be aware that you are the adult now and that you are just using thoughts to remember some events or situations, they are not your reality now. They are memories from your past. However, what can help is if you can use your imagination to see yourself as the child in the third person and embrace, hold and nurture them, as they would have needed at the time.

THE MAMMA COACH

Visualise telling that child what they needed to hear.

Love them unconditionally.

Show them the loving kindness that they may long for if they need space and ideas to heal. Then, step back into your adult self in the present moment and write down what you comes up for you instantly.

Know that this is a healing process and take from it that you will do what you can to ensure your new child has their emotional needs met as much as possible.

Write what you can, and choose to go back and hold that inner child as many times as they need, possibly for the rest of your life, and that's okay.

Again, this process can be triggering, and it may be useful to ensure you have someone nearby, or at the end of the phone, or see a therapist who can facilitate this in a non-judgmental, safe place.

A note on unwanted thoughts

The reality is that we all have thoughts that stop us in our tracks and make us wish we hadn't had them. They can crop up when we least expect it, or when we are feeling very stressed and pushed to the max.

These thoughts are there as a warning bell.

Our minds are trying to keep us safe and sometimes that not in the most logical, easy to understand way. Or sometimes these thoughts are there out of desperation to end our pain or suffering.

These thoughts can lead to us feeling guilty or ashamed or like we are the only one who has ever had them. Please know this is not the case. Having thoughts doesn't mean we are going to act on them. A thought is just a thought. However, if these thoughts lead to feelings and further thoughts of acting on them or harming yourself or your baby with intention, then it's time to reach out and tell someone.

Rest assured, the majority of us don't act on them. It can help to stop and recognise the thoughts for what they are. And perhaps do some detective work as to why you might have had them. If you can be an observer of them, rather than dive in too deep, you'll find they will pass. If you can, allow the thoughts to be there without trying to dismiss them or push them away.

If they are too shocking, please know you are not alone.

Having intrusive thoughts does not make you a bad person.

Normalising them can be very helpful and talking to others about them if you can. Naming them can also help.

For example:
"Oh hi there, I see you, just another wicked thought, not a nice one, a shocker actually, but still, just a thought."

Dr Caroline Boyd has a website that explains unwanted harm thoughts if you wanted to do some further reading and understand why we have these thoughts, especially in parenting.
Website: https://drcarolineboyd.com/infant-related-harm-thoughts

"Sometimes you just need to talk about something - not to get sympathy or help, but to kill it's power by allowing the truth of things to hit the air."

Anchors

An anchor can be and mean many things as long as it creates a learned response to something. For example, if you leave your keys hanging by the front door, you know that as you leave you are usually anchored in your response to glance up and take the keys off the hook as you leave the house.

Another common anchor we are conditioned to is brushing our teeth at night - there is usually a trigger that automatically enables us to respond and do the thing we are anchored to do.

Another angle of anchoring is a way of grounding an emotional response. The way we respond to emotions is a learned response.

Yes, we were born to externalise our emotions when we need them attending to, but we also learned subsequent ways to repress them internally or other external responses such as shouting.

To keep it simple, there are a few examples on the next page of emotional anchors that can help you in your everyday lives and contribute to your self-care practices or when you are around people or situations/places that bring up unpleasant thoughts and feelings.

The trick with an anchor is to repeat it until it becomes a more automatic response.

Hand on heart anchor

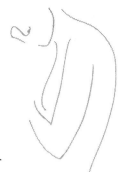

If you notice you feel upset, sad, angry, anxious or fearful, place your hand on your heart or chest and imagine you are holding yourself in that moment.

Imagine you are able to feel safe just from placing your hand there.

Breathe deeply and soften into the feeling. Perhaps notice the warmth from your hand and allow it to soothe you. Perhaps imagine it's the hand of someone who you love very much, holding you and keeping you safe and nurtured.

If you notice a strong emotional reaction about to take over you, place your thumb and middle fingers together on one or both hands and say the words "I am calm, I am safe" over and over again, either silently in your mind, or out loud if you feel uninhibited enough to do so.

Just as an anchor of a boat stops the boat floating away, positive images of places can anchor in positive thoughts and feelings.

THE MAMMA COACH

Self-soothing

Many of us have ways we self soothe that are automatic. We don't need to think of them.

Here are some ideas to help you if those emotions are so strong you need a hug and there's no one around to do that but you. You are able to give yourself a hug, and it will release the hormone for love and bonding, Oxytocin.

Try it now if you like...
- Wrap yourself in a soft blanket
- Cuddle a pillow or cushion
- Have a warm bath
- Apply some foot or hand massage
- Have a cup of hot chocolate or a cup of tea and savor it
- Have a good cry
- Stroke a pet or hug someone else

Now write your own emotions SOS list:

THE MAMMA COACH

Grounding

This is a way of doing what it says on the tin: grounding yourself if you find you are not coping with intense emotions and intrusive thoughts.

In stress response, you can feel agitated, distant, shut down or go on autopilot. This is to keep you safe, however can be pretty unpleasant when it's happening.

Grounding is a way you can learn to bring yourself back down to earth.

Try these ideas out and see what works for you:

- Get back into the here and now by naming the things around you in your environment, saying the date and time, listening to someone talking and what they are saying.
- Breathing - either long and slow or "box breathing" which is in for 4, hold for 4, out for 4 and hold for 4.
- Repetitive movements, such as tapping, wriggling/shaking, strumming fingers, jumping, bouncing a ball, knitting or colouring-in.
- Mindful awareness
- Change environment - Go out for a walk or move into another room.
- Journal - get thoughts out of head and onto paper.
- Get back into your body by pushing feet into the ground, stretching, holding your own hands, pushing your backside into a chair and stomping your feet against the floor.

THE MAMMA COACH

Language & Affirmations

I allow my tears to flow when they need to

I release the emotion I am feeling

I wrap myself up in love and affection

I am held

I am loved

I am secure

I am safe

I allow myself to feel - it's real to feel

Tears are a brilliant release

I let it all go

Crying is part of healing

My heart is healing

I name my emotions and sit with them a while

Tears give me strength to carry on

I hold myself in this moment

I soften into this moment

My baby and I are one

My babies cries are their way of communicating their needs

This will pass

I cherish my inner child

I wrap my inner child up in the love and understanding they need

I give myself the emotional connections I may not have had

I can heal and move on from the past

I choose to stop the past from interfering with mine and my babies future

Write some of your own...

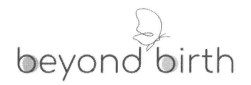

beyond birth

Connections

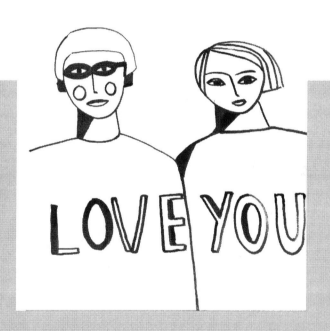

"The energy that
exists between
people when they
feel seen, heard, and
valued; when they
can give and receive
without judgement;
and when they
derive sustenance
and strength from
the relationship"

- Brene Brown

THE MAMMA COACH

Humans are neurobiologically hardwired for connection

This is how a baby is made, born and brought up. As Humans we crave it. We need it for survival, for healing and for inspiration. Without it, we fade away.

I believe later pregnancy and early parenting are one of the best times to reflect on "life-connectivity", and the who's, what's and where's in life as it is presently.

It's a great opportunity to slow down and take stock of who and what matters to us and what we can move on or away from for good or just a while, until we can think and feel in a more balanced way.

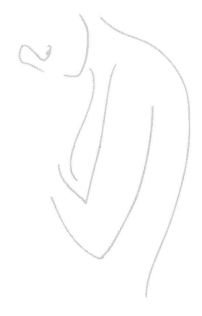

Babies affect all of our relationships

However, a pregnancy occurs, the fundamental thing we all desire is that we are connected and in love with that baby, and also with our loved ones.

Naturally, many lightly contemplate how a new baby will affect their immediate relationships, but wouldn't go any further than that.

Usually because they don't want to dig up old dirt or raise awkward questions or even think about it at all.

What makes us happy and healthy as we go through life? As Mark Twain said:
"The good life is built with good relationships."

Of course, a baby can bring so much love and joy to our relationships, however, many people can be unintentionally in denial of the effects having a baby will have on their lives, and with couples living in more isolated circumstances without an immediate family/village to hand, there's even more reason for people to hope they will be fine - because they know they HAVE to be, but many are not.

What we are seeing is people ignoring the realities when questions are raised and popping their heads in the sand. It's a classic avoidance tactic. If you don't think about it, the potential problem isn't there. But for many, the buried issues can come back in a big way when a baby comes into the picture.

THE MAMMA COACH

Being exhausted, at our most vulnerable and adjusting to a new way of life can bring out our demons, and doing it alone, or without much support can be the thing that brings our relationships to their knees.

It's also important to note that everyone's experiences are unique to them; never more so than during childbirth. What one person felt was wonderful, may be the others nightmare. This may put added conflict, confusion and stress onto a relationship after a baby is born.

"It is ironic that our modern way of life itself involves putting the chief carers of babies under enormous stress themselves." - Sue Gerhardt, Why Love Matters

Isolation and total responsibility coupled with the unrealistic expectations that modern living and society put on us, can lead to feelings of anxiety, failure, low self-worth, hopelessness, and loss for a life that once was or an ideal that isn't matching up to the expectations we hoped for.

This is why it's more important than ever to reflect on our relationships with our loved ones, our friends, our work and vitally, within. The relationship with ourselves is where our resilience lies.

If we can nurture ourselves, we are more likely to be able to ask for help when we need it and ironically, as a result, people may be more attracted to us, thus offering the help where and when it's needed.

THE MAMMA COACH

Choose honesty over perfection, every single time.

Another aspect of this is honesty. Relationships are built on honesty and parenting requires us to address this from every angle. To talk about the good, yes, but also to talk about the bad.

The intrusive thoughts that pop up and make us feel dreadful "Where on earth did that come from? Am I going mad? Best not tell anyone".

We have to take the rough with the smooth. Life is about ups and downs.

It just isn't possible for everything to be good all the time and our minds are used to dealing with this to a certain extent.

What happens when we become parents though, is that we can set our expectations high, because we believe in the dream and this is when intrusive thoughts and feelings surface. When we are under stress our mind clicks into self-preservation mode, and although we instinctively wish to protect our baby, when the stress hormones are released, we react as if we are under attack.

Sometimes that feels like we want to run away, sometimes we have an urge to hide, and other times we feel anger and that fighting urge kicks in. This is normal.

It's just unfortunate when it appears towards our babies or our loved ones. Importantly, most people don't act on these impulses and urges. However, some people do, which is why it's vital we learn techniques to calm ourselves and reach out for help if we feel we will act on our worst fears.

If we can't see eye to eye let's try heart to heart.

So what can we do about this?

How can we take steps to help our relationships stay knitted together?

- Talk
- Listen
- Question
- Reflection
- Touch
- Be loving
- Show kindness and empathy
- Be compassionate
- Lower expectations
- Be honest
- Smile
- Share the load

I've included some additional questionnaires in this guide (see section 8) and ideas that will help you to expand on this and connect/reconnect in a way you may not be used to.

Take your time with them. You may feel just answering a couple of questions at a time is useful, or reflecting on them and saving them for a later date when you are less tired and able to address any issues. Just following the points above should be enough for now.

THE MAMMA COACH

Affirmations

I take time to listen to my partner

I know this time is challenging for us both

We are in this together

We are a team

My needs are not greater, they are intense to me in this moment

What doesn't kill us makes us stronger!

Honesty and communication are key

We ride the ups and downs together

Resentment breeds bad feeling

Love grows love

I grow with you

I slow down and allow myself space to grow

I am aware of my needs and I allow myself to meet them

The softness of your skin on mine brings so much love

I connect with my heart and with my true self

I notice you. I feel you, hear you and see you.

"When emotionally or physically hurt, the touch and closeness from people who hold and comfort you will provide the best remedy. In fact, it has been shown that the same area of the brain is activated whether you have physical pain or mental pain"

- Kerstin Uvnäs Moberg, 'The Hormone of Closeness'

Oxytocin

Oh how I love that we have this hormone!

I'm honestly addicted to it and make sure I get "my fix" every day. My kids and husband are stroked, hugged and kissed regularly. I also love to trigger this in my friends and family as often as I can - rather selfishly, if they get it, so do I!

This beautiful, euphoric hormone produced in the hypothalamus in our brain is pure magic.

Its job is to enable us to feel bonded, connected and loved. It's the "glue" of relationships and helps keep them more permanent.

Known as the shy hormone, it likes to emerge in safe environments, whereby it's not being heavily observed. Helpful in the bedroom, it aids sexual desire and climax, but only fully when we feel uninhibited. It plays the lead role in childbirth, being responsible for uterine contractions, the detachment of the placenta and then triggering the mother's milk let-down reflex. It helps (along with Prolactin), a mother and father/partner/caregiver to bond with baby and baby to feel safe, secure and nurtured.

It helps to induce a sense of calmness and makes a parent feel good, less stressed and more relaxed. The baby also feels good affecting parent and child connection, building trust and love.

Simply put, the more oxytocin we stimulate, the more we want, because of how it makes us feel "loved-up" and needing more where that came from. We can, as I am, become addicted to the source of oxytocin, which is nature's way of keeping us together.

THE MAMMA COACH

The science of falling in love

Triggered in many ways, oxytocin is released via the blood, and the nerves. It also has the power to diffuse into other areas of the brain and organs that affect wellbeing, calm, pain sensitivity, stress hormones and heart rate.

The power of touch and having skin to skin contact actually switches on the "rest and digest" body programme which lowers stress, enhances digestion and healing.

The parents' skin temperature raises to keep the baby warm, reduces the baby's energy-requirements and improves blood sugar levels. It also imprints safety for the baby and enhances the mothering instincts.

So much needed at this time, basically, the baby and parent become one.

This contribution to brain development continues to benefit as baby and child grow as the parent consistently provides support and a loving presence, especially in times of upset and anger, helping to regulate the emotional states, as the infant and child brain is wired.

THE MAMMA COACH

Write down the last few times you have felt the oxytocin hormone in your body and what it's felt like to you.

What can you do to increase the oxytocin flow in your life at the moment?

THE MAMMA COACH

"In the first year, our babies expect to be physically close to the mother as primary attachment figure and, with time, to participate in an increasingly complex social environment that grows to include father, siblings extended family, and friends."

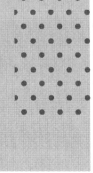

Attachment

Babies are hardwired for care and to learn from their environment and whoever is primary carer. It's usually the mother initially, but obviously, not in every case.

Ultimately, a baby will become attached to and learn from them, triggering emotional and social learning within the areas of the brain affiliated with relationships. This basically builds solid attachments and leads to balanced emotions in the limbic brain, all via positive interactions such as smiles, eye contact, laughter, joy as the baby mirrors the behaviour of the parent - on a psychological level too.

On the flip side, babies can't regulate their own emotions, so they can get easily overwhelmed by feelings of fear, excitement and sadness. They are attuned to the parent's moods, so it's often sod's law that if you are having a low day or two, baby will be in sync, which can make life tougher, and if the parent is emotionally unavailable babies can become highly stressed and it can result in being a vicious cycle.

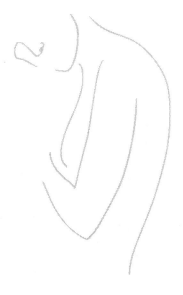

THE MAMMA COACH

Attachment is as central to developing a child as eating and breathing.

With secure attachment, a baby will develop good oxytocin function, giving them a way to be calm and connected faster when under stress.

Once a bond is made, just thinking about a loved one can release oxytocin.

Sensory memory can be triggered and lead us to feel loved and calmer, but as we know, sometimes we crave that physical closeness and need a good hug to satisfy us!

The same goes for adult attachment.

Top tips to help with attachment and attunement:

- Skin to skin
- Conscious breathing
- Grounding
- Sling carrying
- Cuddles
- Eye contact and face to face mirroring
- Sensory memory
- Visualisation of our loved one - or photos to hand
- Voicing our love to someone
- Socialising and friendships
- Trust and honesty

Loneliness and detachment

Having a new baby can feel lonely after the first few weeks, once the events of the birth and bringing the baby into your arms has settled.

Feelings of being detached or isolated from the world as we knew it often kicks in once our partners return to work, and/or family members and friends resume their lives, possibly some distance away.

It can feel quite a shock to the system to slow down so much, and our minds have been used to being full of work and a long 'to do' list. This can lead to feelings of anxiety and restlessness as we learn to navigate a very different list of things to do or not to do, and life is generally slower and dare we say it, quite boring.

So, with the potential boredom comes questions from our inner critic, especially when we are tired, we can focus on the things that we feel we are not getting right, and for a new parent, that could be a lot, because expectations and hopes are high and the reality is often far from what we imagine it will be.

THE MAMMA COACH

We all feel it

One of the best ways to counter this is to do things for yourself that you love to do or that give you pleasure or bring about good feelings.

Nothing grand, and something you can involve your baby in or do while they are asleep. Set yourself small tasks. Keep occupied in a way that fuels you - not just watching TV all day or scrolling through the social media posts of everyone else that looks like they have it together and are doing everything better than you... that will be a sure way to tip your mental state out of balance.

Be kind to yourself and realistic.

If you find socialising hard, then don't go trying to make loads of new friends in the local park. Perhaps join a local Facebook group first and if you connect with someone there, then make an arrangement to meet them and take it from there. Calling friends and loved ones is a great way to feel connected too and you may well make someone's day by picking up the phone and asking them how they are.

As your baby gets older and you get to grips with their feeding/sleeping routine, you may find it easier to venture out to a group or two. However, don't force yourself unless you feel it will do you good.

Sometimes a lot of stimulation is too much for a baby and you. If you miss work, then think about what you can do to feel like you are still utilising your brain power. Again, nothing grand, just small steps to help you feel like you are actively doing and achieving something.

So, how can you fill the void if you feel one?

What can you see yourself doing if you sense this detachment or loneliness kicking in?

Can you reframe these thoughts and feelings?

Write a bullet point plan or ideas on what you see yourself doing and make a pact with yourself that if and when you notice this creeping in, you will do something from your list to reconnect again.

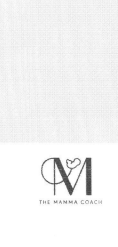

THE MAMMA COACH

Affirmations

I take my time to slow down

This time is unlike any other time in my life

This feeling will pass

I take time to connect with my baby

I use my senses to be more aware of my environment

I use my senses to absorb myself with my baby

I bank this time I have so I can reflect on it later

I fill my time with connection to myself I recognise that

feeling lonely is a sign for me to reflect on why

I use my time wisely

I reach out to friends and family when I feel lonely

I attune to the feeling of connection

I take time to reach out to others

I allow myself to be and feel loved

I nurture the relationships in my life

I move away from those that don't make me feel good

I cherish my loved ones I love to love

I am kind

I am loving

I allow others to like and love me

Endorphins

These feel-good hormones are our natural pain relief and de-stressors which also enable us to feel euphoric, especially when coupled with Oxytocin. Thanks to Mother Nature, we have the ability to feel really loved, high and pain free if we tap into these magical hormones!

They are triggered simply by:

- Laughing
- Soft stroking and caressing
- Showering
- Bathing
- Swimming
- Exercise
- Sex
- Eating hot peppers and some chocolate
- Music
- Scent (lavender especially)
- Acupuncture/Acupressure/Massage

THE MAMMA COACH

So what are you waiting for?

When was the last time you did any endorphin releasing activity?

What can you fit into your day today?

It might help to be mindful of these buzzy, bio-chemicals next time you do any of the above and really tune into the beautiful glow they give you.

THE MAMMA COACH

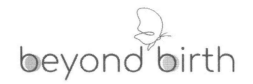

Healing

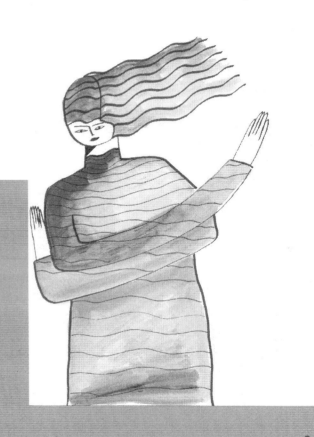

Feel the feeling
but don't
become the
emotion.
Witness it.
Allow it.
Release it.

What are we healing from as we become parents?

Be it the first time or the fifth time. Bringing a baby into our lives inevitably accompanies a necessary time of healing and transformation.

Of beginnings and endings; forgiveness and gratitude; connections and disconnections.

It can be physical healing from birth, even the most straightforward births need time to heal from, or it can be physical and emotional; hormonal and psychological.

Healing comes in so many forms. It could be that as we find ourselves landing into parenting, we witness our mind throwing up distant memories of our own childhood and the questions that brings.

Unfortunately, it's not often the good memories that get our attention (although of course they are there somewhere), but to keep us safe and help us to learn from negative experiences, our mind actively raises the pain from our past in the hope that we can deal with it, learn from it or in many cases, relive the horrors; not always great when you're already feeling tired, low or in the midst of healing from birth.

Rebuild life from within

This is one of the reasons why it's so good to do some emotional and psychological preparation in pregnancy or pre-conception.

To help build resilience, face some of those demons and strengthen relationships. To see what crops up when we are effectively feeling stronger and perhaps less tired, challenged or in the midst of a healing crisis from birth. Creating and embedding new ways of coping when the curveballs and challenges of birth and parenting hit.

However, many people don't do this; out of fear or denial. And of course, most people manage and so they think;

"Why would we need to do any extra preparation? We are already busy enough as we are. We love each other, we will be okay."

Does this ring a bell? So ask yourself this question:
What do I need to heal from and how am I going to go about it?

If it's met with a blank, then great! If it rings alarm bells and your feel resistance or worry kicking in, then now is a good time to take action and talk about it.

Most importantly, having a space where you can feel held and heard should be top of the list.

'The world is
the place
where the
light enters
you'
~ RUMI

Shame and guilt

You may well have heard this but part of becoming and being a parent, is feeling guilty for so much!

We feel guilty about birth, not doing all we wanted to in pregnancy, finding it hard and not knowing what to do in early parenting, and throughout parenting, we have a constant niggling voice inside our heads. That inner critic says;

"You're not doing this right, you're letting them down, you're failing them, you said you'd be this and you're not matching up".

Sound familiar?

Sorry to say this but, our expectations of pregnancy, birth and parenting are mostly pretty inaccurate. This is usually not entirely our fault, as years of being fed images and stories of the 'how it should be' scenarios by the media, social media, family, friends and even experts' books, tends to warp our perception of what life during this time is actually like.

Therefore, we set standards, expectations and aspirations of ourselves, our status and our babies high, resulting in feeling like we are failing when reality sets in hard and fast.

No amount of guilt can change the past

There is a clear thread running throughout life of how unhelpful messages from society and professionals lead to parents internalising the birth experience, blaming themselves and trying to cope without appearing to be struggling.

The combination of feeling guilt, shame, sadness or loss about this experience and perhaps the inability to talk about it often results in psychological issues and a further impact on close relationships. This can lead to a vicious cycle if we do reach out for help, and find that it is not forthcoming, which exacerbates these strong emotional feelings.

When the right support is found, this can be transformed into a positive experience, as we are able to move away from the shame and self-blame following birth, and instead consider the factors which led to the negative or traumatic experience.

If therapy is not what you feel you need, then going to baby groups, joining online chats, or speaking to a midwife/health visitor or friends can really help to ease the load of guilt and shame. As can writing it all down.

Usually by having it explained, rationalised and/or normalised, it's enough to ease the intensity of these thoughts and feelings. Being 'In it together' with our peers and loved ones brings about a sense of community and deeper connection which we need and crave during these vulnerable, transformative times.

THE MAMMA COACH

Affirmations

I am winging it, and that's ok

There is no such thing as perfect

I am doing my best

My love is enough for now

I take each moment and each day as it comes

I take time to listen and learn every moment, every day

I accept what I can't change

I give up the control of what I have no control of

My baby loves me because I love them

Hands up who uses language like 'should', 'ought' or 'must' daily?

How many times do you think it?
And what triggers it?

It can be derived from guilt that we are not doing what we think is the best course of action, or that we are avoiding something.

Procrastination is another way of delaying something we are not keen to do, and this often serves to raise our stress levels if we find we can't push through it. As parents, when we use this language, it's because we are not feeling in the flow or able to hear our intuition.

It can be triggered by comparisons with other parents, hearing advice from people that think they know best (they mostly don't by the way), or from low self-esteem/negative self-belief.

Classic examples of this in parenting are:
- "I really should be getting at least 6 hours sleep a night by now."
- "My baby should be... by now."
- "I really ought to start losing that baby weight..."
- "My mum said baby must be ready to sleep through the night by now."
- "I must be doing ...because the baby advice book said...."

THE MAMMA COACH

These are all common thought distortions. They are often unrealistic, or not true and always contribute to additional fear, worry and stress that we are somehow not getting it right, not doing our best or not winning at life as parents, or in general.

If we are saying this to other people, it's often because we are doing our best to please them, even if it's not heartfelt or genuine.

'Should' statements typically make us feel more hopeless about the situation and can send our self-esteem plummeting.

One of the best ways to counter this habit (it can become a habit), is to notice when we are using the language to ourselves or when speaking to others, and reframe what we've said.

Reframing usually means, to view it differently or change it.

Being self-compassionate, accepting shortcomings and celebrating strengths genuinely helps to prevent the 'shoulds'.

Replacing with "I am" or "I accept that" can be a good place to start.

Write down as many alternatives as you can to any 'should, must or ought to' statements you say or think or others say to you.

Now reframe them.

For example, "I really wish my baby was sleeping more at night, but I accept that this is just the way it is for us at the moment, and I will set an intent to make the most of the quality rest I am getting instead and not compare the amount of sleep we are getting to others."

THE MAMMA COACH

You are responsible for your life

Blame is always an interesting one. We perceive blame so uniquely and it all goes back to our values and beliefs, often in how we were parented ourselves.

This could be a huge topic to discuss, however, for the purposes of this guide, we are going to plant the seed and take a moment to think about it.

How often have you jumped to blame someone if something goes wrong, but deep down, known it may actually have been you that rocked the boat?

If birth didn't go to plan, then most likely, you will be blaming someone or something and possibly very rightly so. Or perhaps parenting is tougher than you expected, and you're more tired and ratty than ever, looking for someone to blame?

In early parenting, blame is pinned everywhere; from partners, lack of sleep to (heartbreakingly) the baby being 'difficult'. Ever since we were born, we have been part of the blame game of life. It's sad but true. It's a fact and part of human nature. It doesn't have to be like that though, and one of the most rewarding things you can do for yourself and teach your baby and child that you can create the strength of self compassion and forgiveness.

Firstly, think of an example where you may be blaming something or someone or perhaps you are being blamed? Or maybe even blaming yourself?

Write this down - it doesn't need to be an essay, in bullet points will do. Doing your best to be as honest and truthful of the situation as you can.

Then, listen, reflect and respond.
By listening, I mean, take it in, as objectively as possible.
Reflect on this. How much truth is there?
Are we second guessing in places where we are trying to find the missing pieces of the puzzle?
Perhaps you could mentally try this when next sitting with a friend who is gossiping to you.

Respond: be the judge but be non-judgmental.
Can you accept what has happened?
What if you were to apply empathy into the equation?
Then self-compassion or compassion towards the person or thing to blame?

THE MAMMA COACH

Finally, can you forgive?

What would it mean to you to forgive?
How can you forgive?
How do you see yourself forgiving? Yourself, or anyone else?
What more do you need to move on?
Can you take a mindful view?

This comes with acceptance, but also with an awareness that when you were so absorbed with blaming, you may have missed the bigger picture.

How does it feel to have got to this point?
How does it feel to know that both the problem and the solution lie within you?

You have it in you to de-escalate this blame and heal it with compassion. Give it a go.

By learning new ways to manage these thoughts and feelings, you will inevitably feel better about yourself, others and you will show your children how to do the same.

Stopping the blame buck in it's tracks. Bingo.

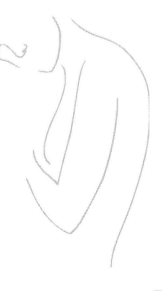

Healing is an art. It takes time. It takes practice. It takes love.

This is a biggie

Naturally, we all need to know that forgiveness is possible.

We all make mistakes. It's in our nature to mess up occasionally and is how we learn, and ultimately, if we fluff up, we hope for forgiveness in whatever shape or form it comes in.

One of the toughest things to do in life is to forgive. Ourselves too.

We are pretty hard on ourselves as we strive our way through our days and nights with expectations of how we should be and what we must do. This also applies to our expectations of others, those we work with, live with and anyone we happen to meet in between. Unless you have a ridiculously stressful job with crazy targets set for you by insane people.

So when things don't go the way we believe they will, we judge, scold, feel hurt, and are thrown off course. Never more so than in pregnancy, birth and parenting.

So, why is it good to practice forgiveness?

Well, it can make us happier. It can improve our mental health, such as depression and anxiety. It can improve our health, sustain our relationships, heal conflict and and increase connections and bonding.

Here are some ways to cultivate forgiveness...

- View forgiveness as something for you, not anyone else. It's to bring you peace and an end to your suffering.

- Express how you feel to others.

- Reflect on the silver lining; what have you gained from the situation?

- If you need the forgiving; make sure it's a good apology.

- Bring empathy into the equation: if you have hurt someone, let them know you are feeling bad too.

- Awareness of the painful feelings is part of the process, so be mindfully aware.

- Humanise the offender/other. See them as nothing but human, with faults like everyone.

- Honestly reflect on what went wrong from or to you. Exaggerating this can dilute the effects.

- Seek peace, not justice.

- Forgiveness is a process. It doesn't just happen overnight.

- If we are resistant to forgiveness, where is this coming from?

THE MAMMA COACH

Compassion & loving kindness

Compassion goes hand in hand with forgiveness. It's where we find the strength to forgive. The base point for it. If we can find compassion for ourselves that's a good place, and from there, loving kindness. If we can, then take another bold step and mentally practice giving those who we have been wronged by the same loving kindness, then it's easier to forgive, and maybe even be grateful to them for the lessons learnt. Easier said than done, I hear you say! Yes. It's not easy and can take time to get there, but as with a mountain, taking the first steps to climb it are the first steps to reaching your goals and a sense of achievement.

Loving Kindness is a practice that can bring about self-compassion and compassion for others. There is a loving kindness meditation included in this guide. It can help to understand what this involves first. The idea is that you first reflect inwards onto the emotion you are sensing and wrap yourself in the loving kindness you need.

Then you reflect that outwards to those you love, then friends, then those you are acquainted with and then the world. This can be very powerful but it does help being guided, so use the MP3.

Once you've managed this, you can see if you can project the same thoughts and feelings towards someone that has let you down or wronged you.

Naturally, this may go against the grain. It isn't easy to forgive people who have hurt us, but it's actually one of the most healing things we can ever do and is usually pretty swift to give us closure on it enough to close the door on it and move on.

What does the word forgiveness mean to you?

How forgiving are you?

Do you forgive and forget easily?

Can you think of anyone you'd like to forgive right now?

Do you find it hard to let go and forgive?

Why is this so hard for you to do?

Write a letter of forgiveness to yourself, to your loved ones and to your colleagues.

You don't need to share this with anyone, unless you feel you'd like to.

Listen to the Loving Kindness mp3 (see resources page for details) and note down how it makes you feel.

THE MAMMA COACH

Affirmations

I am enough

I forgive myself

I forgive others that hurt me

I understand where blaming others will lead to worse feelings for me

I let go of any resentment or anger

I learn from the need to be angry and move on through forgiveness

I let go of any unwanted feelings easily

'I am healing and every day I get a little bit closer to loving who I am"

THE MAMMA COACH

Gratitude

Being grateful is not just about being polite and happy with what you've got. It's so valuable!

When was the last time you were truly grateful for something?

Gratitude practice is a popular and evidence-based way to change the way your mind views things. We can rewire our neurons and pathways to think and therefore allow us to feel differently just by changing the way we think about it.

We learn to be grateful from our own childhood. Our parents or carers teach us to be grateful for many reasons, sometimes to make them feel better for the tasks they do for us, the food they cook for us, the washing, the cleaning, the gifts and so on. In Britain, we are over-zealous with our thank you's, and whilst this is generally a good thing, after a while, saying it becomes meaningless.

True gratitude is said with intent and meaning. If we take things for granted (we are conditioned to do this), then it's worth taking a moment every now and then in the day to stop and notice what we are really pleased about and for.

THE MAMMA COACH

Gratitude

Write down 5 things you are grateful for right now.

1.

2.

3.

4.

5.

Really feel into that gratitude and explore the reasons why you are grateful.

Notice how it makes you feel.

Now try being grateful for something that you wouldn't normally be grateful for. Or perhaps a situation that has happened that you feel the opposite of gratitude.

For example, your taxi doesn't turn up to get you to the airport and you are late for a flight and rush to get there to find it's been delayed. You may not have felt gratitude to that taxi driver at the time, however, you can find gratitude in the fact the flight was delayed and you would otherwise have been waiting for longer at the airport.

What happens if you add gratitude into the equation? What do you notice your mind doing? How do you feel?

THE MAMMA COACH

Affirmations

I am grateful for this moment

I recognise what I have

I am glad you are here

I am glad I am learning from you everyday

I come from a place of gratitude and not from a place of lack

I am able to be grateful for the bad as well as the good

I am learning from every experience and i'm grateful for it all

I take a moment to be aware of all I have and all I am and I'm grateful for it all

THE MAMMA COACH

"Empathy is part of the glue that makes human relationships happen. We cannot survive without relating to others or without sometimes relying upon empathy from others when the going gets tough." - Allan N Schwartz, PHD

As a therapist and coach it's my job to be empathetic. It's part of the therapeutic relationship necessary to form a bond with my clients but also to enable them to feel safe enough to open up and trust me through their healing journey. It's about taking another perspective than our own, which sometimes isn't easy if the situation involves us and we have a differing view. By allowing others emotions to flow, without interrupting until they are ready for us to.

When we are in a relationship, there are many layers of up's and down's, trust and mistrust, intense love and heartbreak, it becomes harder to be truly empathetic. It takes honesty and non-judgement to be empathetic. It requires us to take the non-conditional route being just as open and honest as the person we are being empathetic with.

So if a relationship has been through the mill a bit, then it's harder to feel 100% empathy. That's not to say we can't take an empathetic approach, and this is so valuable as we become parents. Taking an empathetic view with our partners and our children takes practice but reaps rewards as we enable them to express themselves and open up and trust us.

What does Empathy mean to you?

Would you consider yourself an empathetic person? Why/Why not?

THE MAMMA COACH

How can we be empathetic as parents?

How can we be empathetic to our partners and family?

How can you be empathetic towards yourself?

Take a moment to watch this wonderful short animated film from Brene Brown on Empathy Vs. Sympathy: https://www.youtube.com/watch/KZBTYViDPlQ

It demonstrates the value and differences between the two.

This is invaluable when it comes to how we are with each other in our relationships; with loved ones and friends especially.

It also comes into it's own as our children grow and need us to be less directive and more understanding.

Even if the experience you had as a child is raising questions for you as you do this work, it's worth asking yourself how important is it to go back and mourn your past, or be in this moment and choose to take a different path for your own children.

That's not to say your past experiences don't matter; they do very much. It means that for now, you will heal those wounds by changing the cycle of beliefs and behaviors that perhaps led your parents to act as they did.

Affirmations

I take time to listen to others

I take time to listen to my needs

I take time to acknowledge and understand

I know not everyone has the same views as my own

I empathise but I don't take it on as my own

I learn from being empathetic to others and to myself

'The cry we hear from deep in our hearts, comes from the wounded child within. Healing this inner child's pain is the key healing to transforming anger, sadness, and fear.' – Thich Nhat Hanh.

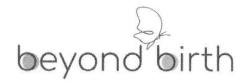

Nourish

Water your own heart, mind, and soul daily; so that you can do, be, and give, from a more nourished and much fuller place.

- Lalah Delia

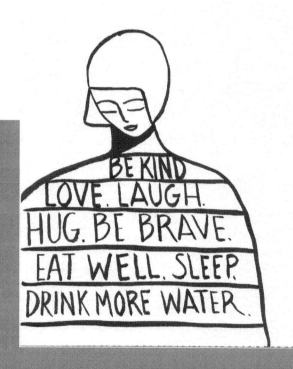

To be nourished is to be content; filled-up, and with energy.

When we see or hear the word nourish, we usually consider food or drink in the first instance. And for good reason. To nourish our body is to stay alive and give us pleasure. When we nourish, we give sustenance to life. We fuel ourselves and top up our resources.

Prior to having children, we most likely had just ourselves to think about, perhaps our partner too. Depending on your lifestyle and what we did/do, staying physically nourished may make it on to the personal priority list.

Maybe you were brilliant at it. Perhaps you were thoughtful about what you ate, went to the gym or a yoga class, cycled to work, dabbled in meditation and met up with friends socially a few times a week.

On the flip side, perhaps you were so busy in your career, that you barely noticed what you were doing when you weren't at work because, well, you were always at work unless you were asleep?

Sound familiar?

Whatever your previous circumstances, and however you reached this point, you may now be wondering if you will ever have a moment to feel nourished in your own right again.

Preparing for and having a baby is mostly all about the baby and the stuff that accompanies the baby; the mountain of material madness that breaks the bank and does little else other than is potentially pleasing on the eye, which is a form of nourishment, and takes over your house pretty swiftly.

It's thrilling in the moment, granted, but can't really do much to help on an emotive level. We often make the mistake and are sold material things, as things that can do the task of helping us on every level. But that's what marketing companies want us to believe and some of us do for a while, because we choose to.

However, not even the poshest buggy/travel system can nourish us emotively, or be a replacement for what we most need at this time; love, compassion, kindness, empathy and SUPPORT.

It may have a good 'support' system' but it's going to do jack for you apart from look good and give you a headache trying to work out how it actually folds down to fit in the car.

THE MAMMA COACH

You've got to nourish to flourish.

As mentioned previously in the nurture section, self-care is a form of nourishment, both physically and emotionally.

It is not selfish to recognise the need for moments of self-care in order to top ourselves up and feel fully nourished again.

Important to note too, that if you find yourself busying and fussing over everyone else but yourself, this is a classic avoidance tactic and can be that you are feeling out of your comfort zone; so take this as a sign to take time for yourself, even if you feel resistant to do so.

Our needs in pregnancy and our needs in early parenting can vary, but they are also similar in that we have a requirement to feel and be nourished.

Our babies are connected to us on the inside and then again on the outside, even if it's not by an umbilical cord. So they need what we need and vice versa. It's all about breath and heart; rhythm and timing.

Biorhythms

Biorhythms are quite complex, but essentially it's about the synchronized heartbeats and natural rhythms of a mother, and later on, father/parent. Like sleep and awake states and hormones like oxytocin and melatonin.

The baby is essentially responding to the cycles of the parent and vice versa.

An interesting fact to note too is that caring for a newborn actually changes parents' brains.

As parents gaze at their newborn; talk gently; use soft, higher-pitched voices; and are positive, warm, and encouraging, their brain's gray matter, or cell bodies, actually grow in the emotion and thought regions that support parenting behaviors.

So, taking time to be aware of and nourish this connection is vital for both parent and baby to feel attuned to each other.

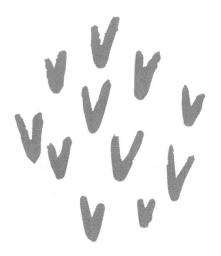

THE MAMMA COACH

In one study, Ruth Feldman, a psychologist at Bar-Ilan University in Israel and at the Yale School of Medicine, observed the heart rates of mothers and babies as they played with each other face-to-face. When the interactions were synchronized in an easy back-and-forth, the rise and fall of mother and baby's heartbeats mirrored each other.

So, in effect, the mother or father/caregiver, helps to regulate the baby's heartbeat through loving, synchronous interactions with eye contact and focused attention.

Feldman noted this is possibly learned by the baby as an "emotional sense of security that accompanies the child throughout life."

Other studies show that oxytocin levels, and even brain alpha waves, follow from parent to baby in harmony too.

So that makes sense when they pick up on our bad mood or tiredness and cry louder and longer. After all that's how we feel isn't it?

In a now-classic study on crying, researchers Sylvia Bell and Mary Ainsworth found that babies whose caregivers consistently responded quickly to their cries, cried less often and for shorter periods of time by the end of their first year.

All the more reason to use tools to lower the stressor hormones and ensure we are engaged with baby when we can so they can mirror this and learn to self-regulate in time.

One of the best ways to learn how to respond to baby is just to observe them as we would do ourselves when tuning into our intuition.

Feeling like we constantly need to do something to attend to our babies needs can be the opposite of what's needed, and often our learning comes from the stillness of observation.

As with our personal intuition; the answers can come when we stop trying and take time to quiet our mind.

Noting a baby's sleep and awake states, their body language and eye contact can be a huge learning curve, but really helps with understanding their unique temperaments, cues and needs.

Task:
Write down 3 things that you enjoy doing:

THE MAMMA COACH

Write down 3 things you can do that nourish you daily

Write down 3 things you can do that nourish you weekly

What can you do to nourish yourself and your baby that will help you both?

What do you notice about your babies cues and needs? Do they do certain things to communicate to you? Is there a pattern or a cycle? Note this down and compare what you see with your partner/loved ones.

THE MAMMA COACH

Noting down how your baby's temperament might change over time is useful.

Note down from birth, then at 6 weeks, then 12 week, then 6 months and a year. How are your emotions and needs changing at these times too? Is there a pattern?

Doing this not only aids your understanding of how your baby is developing, but also how you are managing and the connections and rhythms you have with each other. Know that you are your babies outsourced regulatory system.

Language

Believe it or not, the words we use to others and to ourselves have power. They are everything we know, believe and expect and we can actually physically feel something from a word.

Perhaps you remember the saying or hearing the classic phrase: "Sticks and stones may break my bones but words will never hurt me."

Well, it's not true. Words can hurt. Deeply. And I'm sure we have all experienced this in our lives.

Words act as triggers to feel. So just by suggesting something, we can follow suit by feeling it.

For example; "I allow my head to sink into my pillow" sums up a familiar image of lying down in bed at night and the sensation of our head as it meets the pillow and whatever happens next, perhaps, switching off enough to go to sleep, or triggering the progressive thought processes we have conditioned ourselves to in order to let go of the day.

Words help shape our mindset. They give us direct access to our subconscious where we file all our experiences away and where we attach emotion to each experience.

So by changing the words we use, we can change our beliefs and therefore the emotions attached to the experience. This is how hypnosis works. We bypass the critical mind and go deeper. Using suggestion (words), visualisation and feeling, we're able to make changes at a deep level. Basically, updating the previous version with a new, more believable one. Hopefully that enables us to address any problems as they arise. Words are magic if we allow them to be.

THE MAMMA COACH

"Words are singularly the most powerful force available to humanity. We can choose to use this force constructively with words of encouragement, or destructively using words of despair. Words have energy and power with the ability to help, to heal, to hinder, to hurt, to harm, to humiliate and to humble."
- Yehuda Berg

Affirmations

"I nourish myself to heal and grow stronger"

"I nourish my baby and my baby nourishes me"

"I know I am doing what I can"

"I take care of myself so I can care for my baby"

"I nourish my senses to connect with my baby"

"I take time to myself to nourish my mind and my body"

"I am aware of what I need to nourish myself"

"You nourish me"

THE MAMMA COACH

The power of our senses and being Mindfully Aware

We can get so much nourishment for our mental and physical bodies by tapping into and using our 5 senses:

SOUND

SIGHT

TASTE

SMELL

TOUCH / FEEL

Use your senses now to notice the environment around you and note down what you experience.

Sound can be healing for the soul

What we hear, goes into our thalamus in the brain; the gateway to our consciousness, where it has an impacting effect on our memories, how we feel and what we think about. So much research has gone into the power of sound and music in terms of how we can use it to heal ourselves and others.

Some sounds are soothing, like the sound of falling rain or a waterfall for instance, and other sounds can stir up heartfelt emotions depending on when we heard them before, or just the tones and vibrations of them that resonate with us deeply.

What we listen to is important when we are in a vulnerable state, so you may find that listening to songs about heartache and breaking up with a loved one either helps or hinders you when you are also experiencing a relational breakdown with someone.

Music is magic

When you have a baby in your arms or sharing the room or car with you, think about the sounds you are introducing them to; if you're into punk that may be great for your tension release, but your baby may find it abrasive or they may also love it because you do!

Young babies love white noise, possibly because it reminds them of being in the womb; safe and lulled.

So have a think about the sounds you can play around your baby that will help them - obviously it will affect you too, so having the vacuum cleaner on for hours may not be conducive to you being in a relaxed state even if baby is!

If you can't stand the thought of white noise, then remember that babies love the sound of your voice too. It soothed them in utero and it will do the same in your arms. You may not like the sound of your voice, but they adore it. Think on how you can use that to your advantage and play on the tones of your voice to help your baby sooth or smile. You may feel strange singing to them at first if you're not used to that, but after a while it can become quite therapeutic - even if you just repeat the same easy tune. I used to spend ages softly singing "Frere Jaques" over and over again it and it worked a treat to send them to sleep.

When you are able, being mindful of the sounds around you in your environment is a great way to absorb yourself with the moment and allow the sounds to improve your mood and feelings.

THE MAMMA COACH

What are your favourite sounds?

What soothes you and what stimulates you?

THE MAMMA COACH

Take a moment to tune into the sounds around you right now.

Think about where you can hear them and hear the sound as if you are hearing it for the first time. Absorb yourself with it for as long as you can.

Notice how you feel.

Choose some soundscapes of water, birdsong, rain etc., to play on a speaker in the room.

Close your eyes and take yourself to the place you can hear using visualisation.

Notice how you feel when you are there.

If you have a baby, then notice how the sounds affect them and the sounds they make.

Talk to them about the sounds and explain what they are.

Enjoy x

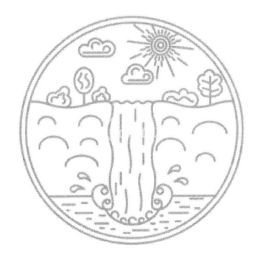

THE MAMMA COACH

The joy of sight

If you are lucky enough to be gifted with sight, you will know the joy we can get from what we can see every moment of every day.

Our minds can see even with our eyes closed, and that's called visualising.

We can have so much fun visualising what we choose to and if we combine visualisation with listening to suggestions, we can really enhance our experience and pleasure.

The mind body connection is incredible when we notice it's power and I'm sure you can think of a time when you've visualised something and really felt it. It's called a psycho-somatic response. We think a thought and our body responds by feeling.

This can be very beneficial for anyone who is struggling with negative thoughts, anxiety and fears. Just by imagining a safe place to visualise (and using the other senses of smell, sound, touch and taste), we can teleport ourselves away from the situation that's making us think and feel in a way that isn't serving us well.

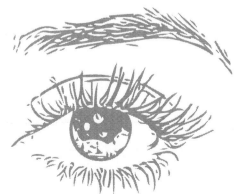

THE MAMMA COACH

What do you like to see?

Look around you for a moment and notice your environment.
Then close your eyes and think about it in detail.
See if you can totally absorb yourself with what it looks like;
the shapes, textures, colours or just a snapshot.
Stay as focused as you can for as long as you can.
When your mind wanders, just bring it back again.
Then open your eyes and relax your concentration.

Now try doing that with somewhere you love to be or perhaps a place you have always dreamt of going to?

See it in technicolor if you can.
Don't worry if you are finding this difficult to do. If you are unable to actually visualise it, then write it down using descriptive words.
'See it' on paper instead.

Set an intent to bank these visuals.

Allow yourself a moment or two to have fun with it and tap into your inner child, the one who lives in the amazing imaginary world.... Just escape for a moment or two.
Nourish your sense of sight.

Think for a moment about what your baby see's day to day.

Depending on their age, your baby is experiencing and learning so much through every sense. Being mindful of our own experiences and also help us to connect with our baby and nourish their experience by tuning into our own and how it is for them.

Poetry by Karen McMillan

That First Year
The year that two became three
No. More. Hot. Tea.
The year of not leaving your side
For more than an hour
And feeling revived
From a two minute shower
The year of white noise
Cuddles and baby slings
As you slowly adjust
To the outside things
The year of sleep regressions
Monkey impressions
Panicked Google searches
Too many to mention
The year I realised that women
Really do hold all the powers
Rocking and pacing
For hours and hours
Being more selective of
The company I keep
And dreading that question
So how does he sleep?
The year of building
All the rods for my own back
Binning the baby books
And not looking back
Endless walks with the pram
To help you to nap
Pounding the pavements
Looking like crap
One whole year to realise
That there's no wrong or right
There's what works
What you need

In the middle of the night
The year of doubts and fears
And bending the ears
Of family and friends
He'll sleep eventually
But when?
But you're more than
Your sleep struggles
So much more
You're that look of wonder
At a knock on the door
Your giggles
Your protests
And that tiny roar
Beaming with pride
As you take in your stride
Learning to roll, crawl and stand
And wave your wee hand
A sudden respect for those
Who've done all this before
But with two, with three, with four
Or more
The year of grand plans and dreams
Of these homemade cuisines
But some days just called
For eggs, chips and beans
And yet somehow you thrived
And we just about survived
The hourly wake-ups,
And some almost-breakups
You really did shake-up
These two kids

Karen hopes her poem inspired you and you can find out more by following her on Instagram @mother_truths. Her books, "Lessons" and "Mother Truths" are available to buy.

THE MAMMA COACH

Poetry by Kate Thirlwall

Perspective shifts

You never listen
I'm constantly listening
You never hear me
I'm trying to process everything you tell me
I'm not important anymore
You're the only person I think about
What do I do?
You look after our baby
But what do I do?
You mother
What does a mother do?
Love.
Love?
It's instinctual. Easy.
Use my instinct?
Yes. Gut feeling.
But my gut has been gutted.
Just trust yourself.
Who do you trust?
Yourself.
My new self? Old self?
Your whole self.
It split open when I had him.
Put yourself back together and walk forward.
Walk on four legs
Yourself.
Two selves.

Gratitude

You work us up.
Broke us up.
Shook. Us. Up.
And then you, and we, remade 'us'.

You made us marvel.
And then two minutes passed and we
would question our decision with guilt
and shame.
You changed our names.
Deranged our claim to freedom.
Brought the new normal.

I fought it and loved it so hard that I
didn't know who I was.
But I was right there.
In a new and old skin I was there.

And time moved us on.
Not on a white charger.
Not in a burst of flame.
Slowly, sometimes glacially it came.
Nature's timeline works counter to the
frenzy of the world.
When you bring us back
You see what you gave up, you see
what seems far away
But then you see what's close
What you chose
What loves you the most
And you can breathe again.
Thank you to my next teacher.
Wiser than grown ups.

Kate hopes her poems resonate with you and you can find out more by visiting her website www.mumstheword.press and by following her on Instagram @mumsthewordpoetry

 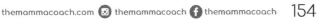

Through poetry we unleash the conscious mind

It can be a sounding board for healing, transformation and growth with the words on paper creatively reflecting the voice of the soul. Creative writing this way can help us be mindful of feelings, thoughts and senses that allow the reader to be present and then to move into another imaginary world, expressing their own relative experiences.

For anyone needing to tell their story and share it, this is an ideal way to do it, subtly hiding behind the words, gaining strength from the reaction of others with every word having meaning and the potential to say more.

I hope her words have an effect on you that helps you to find your way into reading poetry and perhaps writing your own stories this way.

If you wish to share your words or anyone who has inspired you this way, please head over to the Beyond Birth Mindful Early Parenting Facebook Group and get involved.

THE MAMMA COACH

When was the last time you stopped to savor something?

Being busy, we often don't take time to taste our food or drink anymore. Taking time to savor it is seen as a luxury and we are mostly conditioned to think of food as merely fuel, or comfort as a coping strategy if we are emotionally charged.

Our sense of taste is actually primarily governed by our sense of smell, and both are capable of evoking strong reactions both physically and mentally. As the senses have a direct link into our emotional/limbic brain, we're able to remember the things that gave us pleasure and the unpleasant ones.

Generally, we know what we like and what we don't like and get fairly set in our ways in adulthood. Obviously for young babies, it's all new and their senses are highly acute. They are pre-conditioned to be wary of any bitter tastes for protection (anything green and bitter may have been poisonous back in the stone age), and if you're breastfeeding, your baby will be getting some taste from what you've consumed that day, so notice any reactions if you can.

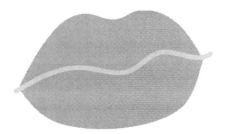

THE MAMMA COACH

Taste Task

Take some of your favourite food or drink and taste it as if it's the first time you're experiencing it.

Savor it and note how it makes you feel.

What images or thoughts come to mind?

When you make your next cup of tea/coffee/hot chocolate, take a few moments to allow it to nourish you.

Enjoy x

Note down your experience:

THE MAMMA COACH

Nothing is more memorable than a smell

We don't give this sense as much credit as perhaps it deserves.

Most people take their sense of smell for granted, but perhaps it will help to know that it's a very sophisticated piece of kit. In-fact, we can distinguish at least **1 trillion** different odors! And unlike the other senses that go via our thalamus in the neo-cortex (our conscious brain), smell has a direct impact on our emotional/limbic brain without us initially being aware. Some smells affect us without us even knowing it at the time.

Every human has a unique scent and human scent affects our brains differently to other scents and more so, our emotions have a scent, which can be contagious!

So if you are around a happy person, then you are more likely to feel the same and that may be down to their smell as well as their giggles. Incredible.

This can also work as a warning system with potential danger or a potential partner.

You smell like love

That new baby smell is undeniably sensational in how it makes us feel - especially our own baby. All the better for bonding with as it promotes oxytocin and endorphin release. Wearing or using scent around a newborn is not advisable for the first 6 months while they get to know and trust the environment they're in, you and anyone familiar caring for them.

It can be overstimulating and block their ability to connect and may confuse and upset them.

I love using aromatherapy, however, would not recommend using it on or near a newborn for exactly this reason because they want to smell you and you them.

If we could bottle that scent, we'd make a lot of money because it's exquisite in how it makes us feel and hugely addictive!

"Listen to your inner voice, because your inner voice might be your nose telling you what to do."
- Johan Lundström, a neuroscientist at the Karolinska Institute in Sweden.

Touch & feel

Ultimately nourishing, even though touch is physical, it has a direct impact on our emotions and mental wellbeing. To touch our loved ones or be touched by someone by way of massage, stroking or hugging is one of our greatest assets when it comes to physical pleasure and subsequent mental calm.

Touch promotes the release of endorphins, our feel good natural pain relievers, and oxytocin, the love hormone. I believe it's our greatest and perhaps most misunderstood sense.

Touch itself appears to stimulate our bodies to react in very specific ways. The right kind can lower blood pressure, heart rate, and cortisol levels, stimulate the hippocampus (an area of the brain that is central to memory).

The physical effects of touch are far-reaching. The emotional effects are mind-blowing.

Without touch, we shut down and fade away. A single touch can affect us on every level from the womb into old age.

It's the first language we learn and the first sense to develop.

It has the ability to heal, de-stress, bond, educate and reassure. It can communicate empathy without words and take away someone's physical and emotional pain. What we feel matters too, so not only what is touching us, but also what we choose to offer ourselves that way.

Wrapping ourselves up in our fave soft blanket is so self-soothing, as is gently massaging some lotion into our hands.

Communicating with our babies this way will give them an emotional sense of security and way of being with others for life; what a gift to give.

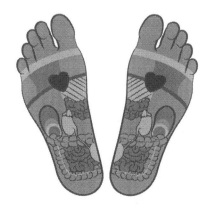

THE MAMMA COACH

Do you like to touch or be touched?

If so why? If not, why not?

How can you introduce more touch/feel into your daily life if you want to?

Sense awareness activity

This activity is to help you practice noticing your sensory experience and by noting down what happens it trains the mind to slow down and be in the moment more - mindful. Thinking about your experience is brilliant but writing it down can really help to imprint it.

SIGHT	SOUND	SMELL	TASTE	TOUCH

Music and sound

Music not only enables us to feel, but it can change our mood and raise memories that take us back to emotive experiences in our loves, or imaginary places we dream of being in. The sense of sound is a gift.

Research for years has gone into the power of sound for healing and proves profound results. Sound heals. It can harm too. So what we listen to affects how we are in the moment by affecting our limbic/emotional brain and triggering subconscious, automatic reaction.

As a singer, and auricular learner (I learn by ear, mostly), I am transformed and soothed by the music I absorb myself in. I find my mood greatly affected by what's on the radio too - my children's choice in music is not the same as mine, so I either tolerate it or subtly remove myself from the room.

Obviously we don't all have the same choices and reactions to music, and that's okay.

Music and sound are able to take your thoughts and feelings to wherever you need them to go and as high, low, comforted or aroused as you like when you truly immerse yourself in it. What a gift that is.

Even those without the use of their hearing can feel the vibrations and rhythm of beats, as can babies in utero. Babies in utero hear and remember familiar sounds and vibrations and are soothed by this when they are born and in the first few months.

When I wake in the morning, I tune into one of many mindfulness meditation tracks which have the option of which sound to accompany the words in each track; I love to hear waterfalls or rain in the background and find birdsong wonderful to wake up to. What we hear when we wake up really can shape our mood for the first part of our day, so be aware of that.

I recently came across a singer songwriter who has used her experience as a mother to write and record some beautiful music and I'd like to share that with you here. Victoria Jane Kearney; singer, musician and songwriter and giving birth to a daughter was the spark that lit a creative fire, leading Victoria to write, record and produce her debut album BIRTH - a memoir of becoming a mother.

Nine songs tell the story of the life-changing journey of becoming a mother. Described as 'beautiful, tender, raw and honest', it takes you on a journey from pregnancy and birth to the intense experiences of motherly love and loss and the deep reconnection with creativity.

To listen to the album visit: https://lnkfi.re/vaHRtLcb

Maternal journal

Creative journaling can support our mental health and wellbeing. Creatives have been using art, words and sculpture to tell their story forever.

It can help us to check in on our feelings, thoughts and put our experiences into perspective. A stream of thought flowing from our minds and transcribed onto paper/screen.

We don't have to be a good artist, or even be able to draw to enjoy creative journaling. Doodling or scribbling will do fine! If the words are stuck, sometimes, just getting anything onto paper is a source of release and subsequent comfort.

Laura, Sam and her team at Maternal Journal have created an incredible FREE resource for people wishing to learn more about the skills and techniques involved in Creative Journaling. In 9 journaling guides, they have given us a way to express ourselves on paper that can be profoundly healing and helpful for our day-to-day mental wellbeing.

Each guide is made by a different artist and designed by illustrator Merlin Strangeway.

You can download all the resources and guides directly from the Maternal Journal website: https://www.maternaljournal.org/

Why not give it a go and share your creations (if you would like to) with the growing private community of Beyond Birthers on Facebook?

THE MAMMA COACH

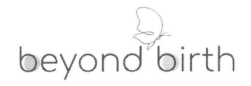
Transformation

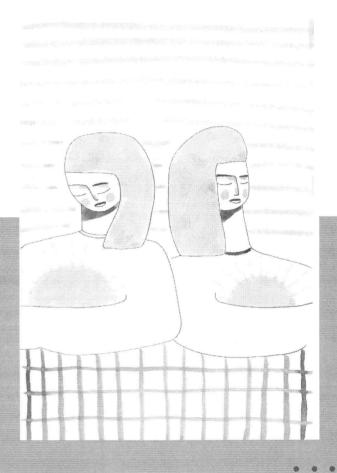

It's not about perfect, It's about effort.
When you bring that effort every single day, that's where transformation happens.
That's how change occurs.

THE MAMMA COACH

I'm a great believer that life is our unwritten book and the significant changes we experience in our lives are just like new chapters.

Pregnancy being one chapter, birth another, and then the baby phase another, and so on.

I adore butterflies, they symbolise rebirth and for a woman, pregnancy and birth into parenting can be comparable to the caterpillar into chrysalis, cocooning, gestating, transforming, to ultimately emerging as a butterfly. Not knowing what colours she will have on her wings.

With birth being the ultimate sacrifice giving life for the mother and the baby at the same time. The birth of a mother and the birth of her baby.

Now, its not my intention to leave fathers or partners out. You are highly significant of course and science has proven how a man's biochemistry and brain changes during this time. For obvious biological reasons, it's a different experience for a man and a woman.

This is a time of adjustment for everyone. Mental adjustment and physical toll. We imagine how we would like to be and how we would like to act in parenting. Be it the first or 4th child, we are often trying to rectify past mistakes or re-enact a positive experience again.

THE MAMMA COACH

The wobbly bridge analogy

It's not easy crossing over.

Some love the challenge and the headiness of it, whilst others find it pretty scary. For all of us, even if we have done this shizzle before, this time can feel uncertain leaving us unsure of what's on the other side and doubting our innate abilities. It's the unknown.

Every birth and every baby are unique. Just as we are unique. But the reality is we all have moments feeling a little anxious of the unknown and that's okay, it's normal and useful to have some anxieties at this time, it keeps us on our toes and ultimately, safer. A bit like wearing a safety harness over that wobbly bridge really.

Enabling us to be more aware, vigilant and wary of our environment, other people and what we do. Some of us find ourselves needing to be bold, finding courage and inner strength to take one step in front of the other. Some days may feel like you want to run back or just can't move on. Stuck where we are. If you expect this, it can make it easier to accept those days and appreciate the days when you feel like you could fly over.

So how do you deal with the unknown? Think back on a time you planned for something big - a wedding perhaps? How did you manage it all? Did you leave no preparatory stone unturned? Were you able to leave it to the gods on the day? Or were you stressed and worried the whole time until it was over and then you felt disappointed or relieved?

Every next moment is unknown.

We have no control over what happens next in reality, but we can control how we act and what we think.

When I teach about birth, one of the things most women say they are afraid of is giving up control. However, in birth, the control is in the hands of the body and we can control our thoughts, relaxation, how we breathe and how we move to assist the body to birth.

The process of becoming a mother: Those physical, psychological and emotional changes you go through after the birth of your child now have a name: matrescence. The process of becoming a mother, which anthropologists call "matrescence" has been largely unexplored in the medical community.

Anthropologist Dana Rachael coined this phrase in the 1970's and scientific research has now proven that the first months through years after a baby is born has similarities to adolescence. The ups and downs of our hormones as they surge and dive, carving out a new balance is similar to the huge changes we go through as teenagers. The mental impact of these changes is also something to consider that is often misunderstood and overlooked. This is pretty significant when you look at life as a whole. This transition is a BIGGIE, and EVERYONE is affected, there's no denying that or shelving it for another day.

Matrescence describes the time from pre-conception through the first year of parenting and beyond. This time affects a mother on every level be it physically, psychologically, socially, spiritually and even politically and economically. Changes for a father or partner are notable too, but considerably less so in terms of physically and hormonally.

THE MAMMA COACH

Emotions

Having contradictory emotions and sometimes irrational thoughts and behaviors are all part and parcel of this time and it's all down to our maternal brain neural plasticity if we are hardwired, or changeable.

Having an understanding of these changes, can help mothers and their partners validate and normalise some of their thoughts and feelings during this time.

It can be a time when you feel low and then high and wonder if you're a good parent or not.

This discomfort is part and parcel and may be talked about with more ease and less shame, if it's better understood and seen as normal.

Obviously, this varies for everyone, and some people do find their mental wellbeing out of balance, leading them to higher anxiety or depression, and it can mean a visit to a professional therapist or doctor to ascertain if this is the case.

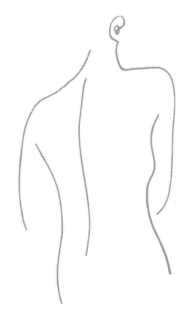

THE MAMMA COACH

If you have any of the following symptoms is could be more than matrescence and if they last longer than a few weeks, then please reach out for more support:

- feeling down and teary
- an inability to concentrate
- feeling worthless
- inability to feel happiness
- anger
- finding it difficult to leave the house
- overeating
- problems bonding with your baby
- suicidal thoughts
- panic attacks
- difficulty sleeping (not due to baby night wakings)
- a sense of dread paranoia or worry about other people
- headaches and tension
- mind overwhelmed and really busy with thoughts
- dwelling on situations and going over them again and again
- restless and lack of concentration
- regular intrusive thoughts of harming baby being more compulsive than usual

THE MAMMA COACH

Being good enough

The phrase "the good enough mother" was coined by British Pediatrician and Psychoanalyst D.W Winnicott. He observed how a new mother is entirely devoted to her baby's needs, often sacrificing her own requirements. Over time, she conditions the baby to wait for longer periods for comfort and food, being just enough but not perfect. This is a careful balance of love and illusion for the baby so they learn not to expect everything their way every time; something that many new parents worry about getting 'right'.

If I had a £1 for every time I thought I'm not a good enough mother or heard this from my clients, I'd be a very rich woman. It's a fact of life that in our society, we have been conditioned to believe that at times (or always in some instances), we are not meeting expectations or standards, be they our own, those of our parents or those of society in general.

Media says that we are not clever enough, fit enough, good-looking enough, brave enough, confident enough, rich enough, funny enough, experienced enough, and the list goes on...

As a parent, it's our responsibility to ensure our children are protected, nurtured, nourished and learn the ways of the world. And with this brings our self-doubt, guilt and shame that we are somehow failing.

THE MAMMA COACH

Our experiences

If our experience of birth was negative or worse, then we will most likely automatically experience some feelings of failure, shame, or guilt. Or perhaps we have to leave a job we loved to become a parent, or we don't believe we are earning enough to support our growing family. If we have a family with high expectations already, then this can add to the pressure or worse, lead to feelings of inadequacy, failure and never meeting the mark. However, even a positive birth experience and a good start to parenting may not be enough if there are ghosts in the nursery or skeletons in the closet. There's a shift in identity that comes with becoming a parent, and if this stirs up some stuff from the past, then get the ball rolling now to avoid any additional stress at a time when you need your mind intact.

Where does this image of the perfect mother come from anyway?

Being a perfect parent is a myth. There is no research or evidence that says that perfection is what our children need. Our children need parents who are fulfilled, connected, present and content. This will look different for everyone.

Saying yes to help from others is such a necessary and powerful thing to do. It takes a village to raise a child. Who is in your village that will allow you to be yourself as you parent but will be there when you need them to be part of yours and your child's life?

There is a great deal of embodied wisdom in our communities that will be useful to you if you can engage with it. Don't expect that you will be able to do it alone in every aspect in our modern society.

THE MAMMA COACH

How we parent matters, and our children will model how we do this for them, so having a greater confidence in our ability to parent and not struggle with seeking a perfection that doesn't exist, will demonstrate to them a more balanced, 'good enough' view.

What does not being good enough look like to you?

List the things you feel this statement is true for you.
Can you reframe them?

THE MAMMA COACH

Affirmations

I am enough

I am worthy

I value myself

I strive for balance not perfection

I am learning every moment of every day

My baby and I learn together

Being a super mum is a Myth

I trust in my ability to parent my baby, my way

I respect my needs and desires so that I can parent

consciously

THE MAMMA COACH

Loss of identity

Becoming a parent can, to some, can feel like loss or grieving, which is hard to realise or admit at the time. It can feel like restlessness or emptiness. Some feel like they don't know who they are anymore. Not just appearance, but also character. Relationships have to open up and it's a complex time of ambivalent emotions and a need for a trust that may never have been there. It can also be empowering, a beautiful period of repair, and growth; greater connection, greater security and realisation of self and love for others you didn't know we're capable of.

A certain level of disconnection from who you were is necessary, like shedding a skin, so that you are you, but a new version of you.

So what does this actually mean? What is this new version of you? It may be a very subtle change, or it could be life shifting. What is usually meant by this is the impact that pregnancy, birth and becoming parents has on us on all levels: physically, psychologically, spiritually, socially, economically and politically.

Pregnancy is often compared to the crysally period or time of gestation; in effect, when the substantial change (or death if you're a caterpillar) occurs, a mother's body becomes the host for a new baby and all that grows and changes with that. The enormity and significance of this is often overlooked, or not discussed, but it leaves some women struggling immensely with just the concept of this, let alone the reality. There are mothers who find themselves suffering throughout and others who glide through without any complaints. We never know how it will go and each pregnancy is different. This has an effect on how a mother (and her partner to some extent) feels about becoming a parent with ambivalent feelings towards having a baby and what it means and all the changes that happen as a result.

Then comes the birth

The birth of a baby and also the birth of a mother (and father if appropriate). However, birth happens, it has a profound effect on us for the rest of our lives and our babies too who are not usually considered significantly until we hold them in our arms. Birth is intense for both parent and baby and if the process was not as expected or hoped for, will have an effect on both for days, weeks, months or years after. This is why it's so vital these experiences are reflected on, processed and understood by parents, as part of their healing and recovery, as well as that of their babies.

I view birth as an emergence. The most profound change we go through in life. Our butterfly moment. Miraculous and profound; leaving an imprint on mother, child and father/partner for life.

Delicate and vulnerable that requires enormous strength and resilience. The only control we have is to allow nature to take it's turns, and if not, then we have medics and machines to do that for us. Birth gifts us a new identity and strips us of our innocence.

Some found they weren't ready to transform and others are more than ready. Some people take years to feel like parents, and others were born wanting to be parents. Where do you sit here?

Our new identity as a parent affects mothers or the main caregiver mostly. A father/partner is better able to 'wear two hats' if they are leaving the nest to work every day. Although this may be gut-wrenchingly hard for some. A mother may feel resentment of this as she can feel suffocated by the constant groundhog day demands of caring for baby and maintaining the nest. She may also love her new role, especially if the work she did before was not making her happy.

THE MAMMA COACH

Parents can feel trapped by parenthood

It's important to notice that when it starts to creep in. Going from 2 to 3 or 3 to 4 children etc., it can feel to some like they are caged in and the urge to escape can be strong.

There is nothing wrong with feeling like this, but if it's becoming a problem, then it's vital those feelings are talked about.

We don't go to parenting school and babies don't come with a manual.

We have to find our feet and learn quickly with additional pressures in the mix; often less salary coming in, needing a bigger house/car, holidays are not as they were, sex may not be on tap, bodies have changed, priorities have changed and the fun factor has had a revamp.

Adding our expectations of the parents we believe we will become and may not actually be able to match up to, the identity shift can feel like a crisis to some. However, as I mentioned, not everyone will feel like they are failing, some were just born to fly as parents and that we must accept. And not compare ourselves to them if we can help it.

THE MAMMA COACH

Comparison and envy of others

This is an enormous topic that I can only touch on here, but one that comes up time and time again in the parenting society we find ourselves in.

During times of transformation we can feel stuck, or out of sorts. Unable to move forward and longing for our previous life or lifestyle, even the negatives can feel attractive when we are unsure of, or bored of, the life we find ourselves in. We may find ourselves envious of our loved ones and friends if we see them getting on with their lives in a way we are yearning for.

Can you think of any time in life where comparing yourself to others has been beneficial? This may well be possible. We can use comparison to spur ourselves on and get out of our comfort zone to achieve things we may not have believed we could before. This can be advantageous and empowering in the right circumstances and can even help us to understand our status in our relationships and friendship or work groups. We need a level of competition to survive. However, comparison from a place where you are doubting yourself, your abilities or lacking, may be more detrimental to mental balance.

One of the situations we find ourselves in as parents is we can believe that everyone else is getting it right and we are not, when we feel out of control a lot of the time, we tend to look to others and how they are managing and tell ourselves a narrative about them that may not be true. Our inner critic is strong at second guessing and has us believe anything in order to fit together the missing pieces of the jigsaw puzzle, even if it's irrational and untrue. It's a funny way to keep us safe, but that's fundamentally what our mind is attempting to do; and unless we realise in time, it can lead us to think, feel and act in ways that are out of character.

THE MAMMA COACH

Baby sleep

Sleep deprivation can lead us down a rocky irrational path and we may convince ourselves that everyone else is getting sleep and we are not because our baby is tricky/naughty and we were bound to end up with the only baby that doesn't sleep in the world!

This kind of thinking is actually pretty normal for the majority of sleep deprived parents, because their minds are desperately trying to solve the problem. But it's also a lonely place to be, having us think we are the only ones struggling.

Coming from a place of envy, jealousy, comparison, insecurity, low self-confidence and selfdoubt is a dangerous cocktail for any parent. It can have a huge impact on our mental health and our relationships. Being vulnerable as a new parent is generally when these issues can raise their ugly heads, so being aware of this and taking precautions/preparing, can help to minimise the demons.

For instance, coming off or taking a step back from social media, only having friends and family around you that make you feel good about yourself, being realistic and authentic with yourself and others and asking yourself "WHY?" and "Is this realistic or true?", when those thoughts crop up.

There will be times when we wish we had a magic wand; for someone to tell us how to do it, what to do, or just to be able to know ourselves. This is a time when comparison of others in a similar situation can feel strong, especially when we have people telling us how they would do it, or reading the books leaves you feeling even more helpless and overwhelmed than before you read them. These are times to take a step back from trying and comparing and ask yourself what your gut feeling is saying, and what you would say to a friend in your shoes. Sometimes, stopping the noise and taking a more proactive, problem solving approach can pull you out of the quagmire and help you feel more in control again. People who feel in control rarely compare themselves to others.

Building your self-confidence is one sure way to help defend yourself from the envy demons, so here are a few questions you can answer that may help tip the scales in your favour:

What are your positive characteristics?

THE MAMMA COACH

What are your values?

What do you believe in?

What are you good at?

What are your negative characteristics? Why?

What don't you believe in? Why?

What are you not very good at? Why?

What makes you happy?

What makes you sad?

What are your aspirations?

What are your expectations?

What is your chosen parenting style (do you have one?)

Does any of the above matter? Why?

THE MAMMA COACH

Does this matter to others? Why?

Write any additional thoughts here:

Ambivalence is a state of having simultaneous conflicting reactions, beliefs, or feelings towards some object. Stated another way, ambivalence is the experience of having an attitude towards someone or something that contains both positively and negatively balanced components. The term also refers to situations where "mixed feelings" of a more general sort are experienced, or where a person experiences uncertainty or indecisiveness. (Wikipedia)

The push and pull of parenting. Why am I including it in this guide? Mainly because parenting is so ambivalent.

We love it and we hate it.
We need it and we want it to go away.
We take pride in it and we feel like we are failing.
We laugh and we cry.

I could go on and on.

Understanding this about parenting can help us to take it in our stride and take the rough with the smooth; to lower expectations and accept that there will be good times and blinkin' awful times.

Ambivalence exists in the space between our expectations and the reality of parenting. It can make us feel like we are nailing it or failing at it and often comes from a place of fear, uncertainty and avoidance.

THE MAMMA COACH

List your ambivalence in parenting or pregnancy, or what you imagine will bring on ambivalent feelings in parenting.
Note what you might do about this, if anything?

This may help to problem-solve the strong negative thoughts and feelings that crop up and help to understand where they come from and why they are there.

If you note that you are siding more on the negative when you think of your ambivalent feelings. This is quite normal and if you can notice what comes up for you it can help you.

Perhaps it's a strong resistance, avoidance or you may have a strong urge to resolve the feelings. That's also very normal. Ambivalence is not a comfortable place to sit for long and we often lean in one direction or another.

THE MAMMA COACH

So, if you can, note what comes up for you and see where it takes you.

For example: you know you love your baby very much, but they have colic and cry so often that you can't stand the noise and want to run away or make it stop and you can't so it makes you question your feelings and the thoughts that may appear as a result of this situation.

Can you think of any affirmations you'd like to add here?

Movement

Even though this guide is about the mind elements of early parenting, we would be crazy not to mention the affects that movement or lack of, has on our mental wellbeing.

The mind and body are connected and when one is not functioning well, the other follows. Through movement, our bodies thrive. We can feel more alive and alert. Have more clarity of thought and take satisfaction from knowing and seeing how our bodies respond.

However, I am a firm believer in moving the way we feel our bodies want and need to move. Especially in the first year of parenting. Gentle movement like walking, yoga and pilates are highly recommended due to the subtle, effective results they have on tone and mental balance.

They bring us in tune with our breathing, how our bodies feel and help us to be aware of the healing we are going through. They can lift our mood and in the case of walking, put us in touch with nature and all the benefits that brings.

Too often, we see people putting pressure on themselves to 'get back to their pre pregnancy body' using extreme dietary and exercise techniques to do so.

This works for such a small percentage of people who usually naturally have the metabolism and physique to bounce back.

The majority struggle and can be left feeling even worse than before, with low self-esteem, body dysmorphia and unhealthy habits that interrupt the recovery they are already going through.

Be realistic. Be authentic. Move how you want to move. The benefits of this far outweigh the fads and the unrealistic images we are sold in the media. If you can learn to love yourself as you are, then you'd be amazed at how much your body and appetite responds. If you love something, you tend to it, care for it and it becomes healthy and blossoms as nature intended. Have a think about that and write down some affirmations you know will help you to find your way

THE MAMMA COACH

"Happiness can only exist in acceptance" - George Orwell

Accepting who we are now is so powerful. As is accepting what has happened to get us to this point, and all that will come as a result of how we live our life and the unexpected. What we have no control over, we must accept, or feel like we are fighting an invisible force that will always win. This is fundamental to parenting.

If we can accept that we can't control others, especially our children, we can watch and learn ourselves. Being accepting doesn't mean lying down defeated. No. It means recognising when we can't win, change or prevent its outcome. As a part of the transitional experience of parenting, when we accept the transformation, we are in effect winning and as a result, enjoy the moments of happiness and contentment that brings. We are what we are. We become who we become. The only control we have over this is how we are and what we learn from our life along the way.

Once our babies are born into our arms, they are individuals. Being conscious to this fact helps us to accept that as much as we hope to mould them into mini-me's or ensure they don't make the same mistakes we did/shelter them from the world, we must resign to the fact that we have no actual control over what's going on for them as individuals, especially what they are thinking. We can teach them, protect them and nurture them, and that is essential. That is pretty much all we can do.

Being accepting of the experiences that have led us to where we are now is so powerful. There is no failure, only lessons learnt, which is tremendously hard to accept at times. It's in our nature to fight anything or anyone that we feel has wronged us, so acceptance and forgiveness don't come easily at times. It takes practice, commitment, motivation and belief to move on sometimes and that's okay.

THE MAMMA COACH

Acceptance of how we are now helps us to heal and notice more of what we have instead of what we don't have.

This mindful practice enables our minds to latch onto the abundance in our situations instead of the lack or longing for more or differing circumstances. Having a baby in our arms, and allowing the connections to grow from how we feel and think often leads to greater acceptance when we tune into what's important to us in those moments. To accept and soften into the moments, rather than trying to change or protest them can be both empowering and give us a sense of peace, much needed as we navigate the early days, weeks and months of parenting.

What is important to you right now? List your top 10 priorities.

THE MAMMA COACH

What do you think you can accept in your life that you may have been resisting before and why?

What do you struggle accepting and why?
What can you do about this?

F.E.A.R
(False Evidence Appearing Real)

A small amount of fear is a normal part of life; it's purpose is to keep us safe. However, we often find ourselves fearing things that are not considered dangerous or generally life-threatening, and that's when it can help to have some resilience and tactics to deal with them.

We don't need to conquer every fear. Choosing our battles can be beneficial in situations where we may not need to face our fears. For example; if you're afraid of bungee jumping, then do you really need to do it and put yourself through the unpleasant thoughts and feelings as a consequence? If you do it, you may be cured for life, or you might just not be and it could traumatise you for life!

However, if you have fears that you really must overcome, then the only way to manage them is to face them head on. Firstly, educating yourself of the facts is an effective way at taking that first leap, and potentially dousing the flames of fear at the first hurdle.

This happens a great deal in the hypnobirthing courses I teach; parents coming in believing what the media and scaremongering stories portray about birth, and leave feeling empowered, confident and looking forward to giving birth.

This is done with a combination of techniques, but an education about how the body works to deliver a baby, and how mindset impacts this, really helps to flip the negative ideas and beliefs on their head.

THE MAMMA COACH

Perhaps one of your biggest fears is/was giving birth to your child. This is very common, and media and history has hyped it up to insane levels. Mostly we see images of women on their backs, legs in stirrups, in agony. Get the picture? I could write an entire book about why this image is wrong and how women generations ago used to look forward to giving birth because it meant they were revered and worshipped for being life-givers. Somewhere along the way (don't get me started), women were disempowered by fear and lost faith and trust in their bodies and minds to birth comfortably and in control - yes, that's how we are designed to give birth.

However, fear debilitates birth and leads to complications and potentially a mother's body not producing the hormones it needs to give birth, so medical intervention is necessary - and it's good that we have that support available when it's needed, but mostly it's this that we see and hear about in the media and through negative birth stories.

Hence the fear surrounding birth and the belief that our bodies are not capable of birth and the pain is too much to bear. It's right to view pain as something to fear. It's awful and nobody wishes it on themselves; but pain is there to tell us something is wrong and needs fixing.

Childbirth is a normal physiological process of the body and if we relax, breathe and move in a way that helps not hinders, and believe our bodies were created to birth a baby, alongside visualisation, love and a safe environment, then we need not experience the sensations of birth as something to fear, more as a part of the mechanics of the body as it births our baby. There is minimal risk in this and therefore, can legitimately lower our fear state. This takes practice, commitment and belief though, and without that, those fears can come back to get in the way and ramp up the pain sensation

THE MAMMA COACH

Thinking will not overcome fear but action will.

One of the best ways to face fears is to create an action plan and imagine how you would cope, imagine yourself coping and then when you are able, to expose yourself to what it is you're afraid of. This can be a slow, step by step process, but it can also reap great rewards.

Our brains have to actually experience the fear in order to extinguish it, so mental imaginal exposure is a very useful tool, leading to actual exposure to the fear. Fears around how we will parent, how our relationships will cope and how we can provide for our children are very common in pregnancy and parenting.

Taking a solution-focused approach to these thoughts as they arise by writing them down and talking about them is a good way to help defuse them and take away the power they can have over us. As with anxiety, by acknowledging it and welcoming it as a source of wisdom to learn from, like: "Ah, hello old friend, I see you're here to teach me something again.", can help to master it, rather than be disempowered by it.

Celebrating our wins and courage up to now, alongside being grateful are wonderful ways to flip the fear too. Rather than thinking "I can't do that because I'm afraid of...", we can use language that resonates with our subconscious emotional brain and say "I felt afraid, but I did it and felt great that I did.".

Noticing when you are avoiding facing your fear because that feeling of fear is not pleasant, so most of us shy away from it, is a great place to start.

Procrastination is a classic signpost of fear.

What are we avoiding doing because we are ultimately afraid of doing it/the unknown consequences and the lies our mind is telling us?

We can teach our brain that it doesn't need to be afraid by habituating it to the fear - that's facing it, rather than avoiding. It sounds simpler than it is, that's a given. But it can be done with proof given. For instance, telling a child not to be scared of the monsters under the bed is not going to work, we have to go under the bed and show them we are fine, and hug them until they feel safe again, to prove to their brains it's ok.

What are most afraid of right now? How can you overcome that fear?

Come up with a plan. Talk to a professional if it's as a result of trauma. Try to keep this exercise as light as you can. We are not here to open up old wounds, more to work with what we are afraid of in terms of parenting and what that means.

THE MAMMA COACH

Intuition and instincts

Becoming a parent will put you in touch with a part of your instincts you may not have known before; that of being protective and having an understanding of another human other than yourself that you are able to automatically know what to do and what not not do for the other person.

This takes practice and for those of us who are not naturally trusting or tuned in to our intuition for ourselves, it can feel alien to be able to do this for another.

That saying "I just wish I knew what to do.", is going to feel and be pretty familiar as a parent. And don't shoot the messenger, but you do actually know what to do, unless it's a medical emergency, etc., in which case you intuitively know you should seek assistance from a professional.

It's just bypassing the noise of other people's advice, past experiences, fears, self-doubt and so on, that puts a wall between us and our intuition.

Actually, intuition is formed on the basis of past experience and knowledge; it's unconscious thinking, so the brain on autopilot. But even if you have never had a baby before, we are instinctively primed to know how to nurture them and if we trust our gut feeling, we are usually right in the solutions we come up with.

So how can we tune in?

Well, if you're concerned you are not able to hear your inner voice at all for whatever reason, then try these ideas:

1: Step back from the noise. Pause and be more mindful in the moment. Focusing on your breathing can help to do this, as can using sensory awareness.

2: Pay attention. So much of our day is focusing on the external, we can learn a great deal from bringing the focus back within.

3: Stop thinking about the problem for a minute and meditate on the outcome. See what your gut feeling is and because your gut and brain are connected via the vagus nerve and that has an impact on how you feel about a problem.

4: Write down what your thoughts are and the pros and cons. Then go for what your inner voice is guiding you to, often it's the first thing that crops up.

THE MAMMA COACH

Listen up

It is a basic human need to want to be heard and it is frustrating and emotionally draining when we don't feel we are being listened to or understood.

Everyone needs to feel their points are validated and they are respected and duly considered, and if this is not happening, we can feel detached, resentful, stuck and our self-worth and confidence takes a tumble.

Never more so than when we are feeling vulnerable, unsure, overwhelmed and stressed: sound familiar?

Listening is a skill that most of us learn when we are children and fine-tune as we grow into our adulthood. If we were listened to, then we can empathise and usually instinctively know to take the time to listen to others. If we were not heard, then we may find it difficult to truly engage in the attentive way needed to non-judgmentally hear others.

As a skill, it can be honed, and importantly, we can gain so much in our relationships with ourselves as well as others when we get better at it, so aiding the process of recovery and deepening connections.

So, by paying attention to developing the skill of listening we can help our own relationships, our mental health and model to our children as they look to us for guidance and fundamentally look for us to allow them to be heard, building trust, honesty and rapport.

What do you know about listening?
What do you need to do in order to listen in a way that allows someone to feel heard?

Mindful listening

Here are a few ideas on how to listen mindfully and fine-tune your listening skills, with others, but also with yourself:

What is it? It means being present - in the NOW.

Focus - tune out and tune in.

Attentive - face the person and show interest.

Non judgemental - put your judgments aside.

Observing - body language, facial expression (yours and theirs).

Open - your mind, your body and your heart - allow emotions to be expressed.

Intent - set an intention to hear what they have to say and truly listen with your senses and empathy, not sympathy at this point.

Aware - be aware of the situation, any bias, and distractions that could prevent you from listening. Your attitude matters as does appearing supportive.

How to practice Mindful Listening using H.E.A.R

Halt - Be attentive
Enjoy - Take a breath and choose to enjoy
Ask - Openness, curiosity and clarification
Reflect - paraphrase, reflect back and write it down if you can.

Words have power

I've touched on this throughout this guide, but the language we use with ourselves and others shapes our every moment; be it verbally, written down or internally. Words have power to heal and harm, help and hinder.

They are what our conscious and subconscious minds use to function, process information and make decisions. How we learn and unlearn. How we attach emotion to experience and how we detach, refresh and update information and experiences.

What we think and say is what and who we are.

As parents, what we say to our children shapes their learning and their security. Babies learn first through touch and their senses before they learn to speak, and it's in times of great need, that we can also take strength from doing just that too; taking it back to sensory awareness to still our chattering minds and find stillness and peace for a few moments.

Your subconscious mind takes up over 80% of all your mental activity; that's your emotions, imagination and all auto body processes, all your memories since before you were born. It's also your beliefs, habits, preferences and instincts.

So when we get lost in the grips of our subconscious as a result of something happening to us that causes a reaction, that's where we are, whirling around in a place that doesn't distinguish between fact and fantasy and it uses the language of metaphor and pictures to communicate ideas to the conscious mind to instruct us.

You have the power to create change

Like a computer system, the subconscious stores the information and the conscious mind is like the software that questions and dictates. It needs language to function and metaphor in the form of visualisation to update and reframe old thoughts and beliefs that no longer serve us.

If we think we are something, then our subconscious can believe it.

So think you are the parent you believe you can be and your mind will act out that you are. Use language that you would like to hear with yourself and reframe the negative thought cycles into more favourable ones, and you will soon notice the difference in how you think and feel and how others are with you too.

What language do you need to change to instruct your subconscious to believe a new, more favourable narrative?

Here are a few ideas to start you off:
"I choose to direct my mind with kindness and self-compassion."
"I am a good enough parent."
"This guide has helped me more than I could have imagined."

Throughout this guide you will see that the language we use with ourselves and others shapes our every moment; be it verbally, written down or internally.

Words have power to heal and harm, help and hinder. Use them wisely.

THE MAMMA COACH

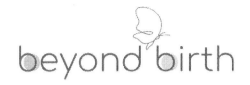

Dads & Partners

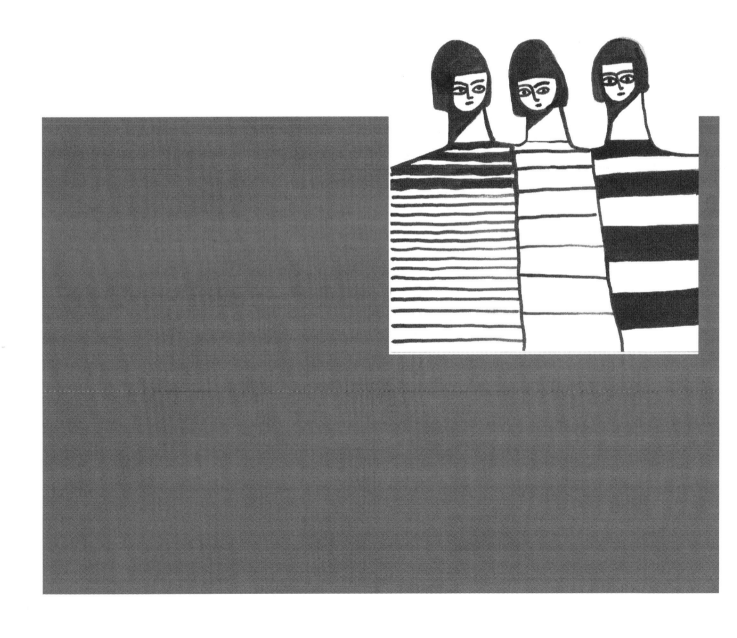

A message from Mark Williams

Founder of Fathers Reaching Out, Campaigner, Author, Consultant and Keynote Speaker on Paternal Mental Health

It's so inspiring to see this pioneering Beyond Birth Guide and Beyond Birth support groups available to all parents that focuses on mental health and wellbeing.

It combines a much needed psychoeducation with simple, tried-and tested practices aimed at helping parents cope with the challenges of the first 1001 days with a baby. Using this guide will inevitably enable more Dad's and Partners to support their mental health and build emotional resilience to protect their mental state, coupled with having a deeper understanding of what their partners emotional needs are.

My lived experience has been beneficial in my work by supporting parents to have an understanding and empathy about the struggles parents entail during the perinatal period.

It is vital that there is trust, confidentiality and boundaries in place for yourself and the parent. Also if you do not have the lived experience your support must be introduced in a non judgement way with empathy with clear understanding that fathers (and partners) can and do suffer during the perinatal period as well.

Fathers (and partners) sometimes need acknowledgement that there are others having thoughts and feelings like they are experiencing which can be enough before it manifests. But there are many fathers who will need that professional help in order to understanding and learn positive coping skills that will be replace the negative ones.

THE MAMMA COACH

A message from Mark Williams continued...

By supporting the father (or partner) it will help support the mother better with her own mental health as well. It will also improve your relationship and your fathers mental health. Many other fathers struggle to bond with their babies and attachment which is important for the development of the child.

Behaviour changes in the perinatal period are very common, for example, substance abuse, anger, avoiding situations, personality changes, physical health problems or undiagnosed disorders worsen.

Triggers for these behaviour changes could happen when fathers or partners witness a traumatic birth, lack of sleep, childhood experiences, etc.. Financial worries, Isolation and previous mental health history can also exacerbate problems.

It is important to have clear pathways for fathers to be supported and engage with specialist services as parents' mental health can be complex.

Sadly we know the biggest killer in men under fifty in the UK is suicide and there is evidence there is high risk in new fathers. A guide and groups such as Beyond Birth can help to prevent a need for specialist help, and also give confidence to reach out to those services if the need is there.

Please see the resources in the back of this guide for further information and support.

Top tips

Life as a couple - There are so many ideas and tools to help in this guide, but most importantly, having an understanding that your relationship will change, possibly for the better, however, with tiredness, birth recovery and now a baby (and all the gubbins) in between you, it will help to be more mindful of new ways to find intimacy and support.

Lower expectations and be super sensitive.

Talk - You may find it hard to talk much, but keep the communication going; keep it light if you can, and remember that laughter triggers an endorphin response.

Closeness - Sometimes, words are not needed. A hug, a smile, eye contact and a handhold may be all that's needed.

Coping - Expect stress and tiredness levels to rise, and your normal ways of coping after a long day, changed. Try to counter-balance this by taking it back to the basic things you enjoy, talking to friends, listening to music, exercise or walking to clear your head.

Connect with your baby; now is a perfect time to have skin to skin with your baby, carry them in a sling/baby carrier, massage or bathe them. Explore their little fingers and toes, the softness of their skin and make eye contact with them as you gently get to know them in your own time, your way.

Maximise **time off** and try staggering your return to work if you can.

More top tips

Expect that you will have **differences of opinion** from your partner, but be prepared to listen to them too. They will be super exhausted and may not be making sense to you, but they will be instinctually navigating a new terrain, there is no manual. Respect that you may disagree over the best path to take at times.

Tiredness and vulnerability can be ugly at times. Expect the worst in this case and it may not be bad at all. Take the baby from your partner and encourage her to rest as often as you can. She may be trying to do it all herself to take the pressure off you, but will get exhausted quickly this way. Try and find a balance for you both. Nurture your relationship and think of novel ways to enjoy time together.

It's the small gestures and the little things that matter. Document this time so you can look back a year down the line and beyond, and feel connected and nurtured again and again.

Eat well - cook or order in nutritious meals and treat yourself and your partner. Now is an ideal time to drop standards slightly, get cosy and shut the world out for a while.

Don't be the hero - if you try to do it all and overload yourself, you will burnout. That's a fact. Also, do your best not to compete with your partner about sleep, or 'me time'. Things can get toxic quickly if this happens. The huge to do list for a perfect everything can wait.

Top tips continued

You may need to drop some of the extra-curricular activities you've been doing to show solidarity/teamwork. Same goes for booze and smoking. Cut back as much as you can. You will reap the rewards in the long run. This doesn't mean stop having fun and seeing friends, but accept the fact it can't be how it was. Your partner needs your support - even if it doesn't feel like it at times.

Find a new bunch of mates - Connect with new parents that have everything in common with you at the moment: a baby!

Recognise your little achievements every day. Come from a place of gratitude and avoid wishing things were different somehow.

This is it. How it is right now. So instead of fighting it, comparing with others, or feeling disappointed in the things that haven't gone how you expected, do what you can to reframe those thoughts and feelings. Be present, aware and in each moment with a sense of gratitude and awe. It helps to write things down when the thoughts and feelings become overwhelming. Failing that, talk it out.

Sometimes **it helps to talk** to a pro, someone who can hold non-judgmental space for you to be heard. You can feel emotionally held in those moments and let go of any pent up worries or fears you feel you can't discuss with your partner, family or friends. Getting support this way is not a weakness, it's a strength and a sensible, caring thing to do.

THE MAMMA COACH

Relationship questionnaire

Here are some things to think about and perhaps discuss with your partner.

How will this baby change your relationship with your partner?

What do you need from each other to find balance? And how will you support each other?

What do you need to let go of? What's holding you back?

Relationship questionnaire continued...

When you are at your lowest, what do you need in terms of emotional and physical support?

How will you cope if the birth doesn't go to plan?

What support do you have around you?

How will this baby change your relationship with your partner?

In laws or out laws?

Whilst we certainly need a helping hand as we adjust to life with a baby, there's help, and then there's "HELP!".

Being aware of how sensitive a mother is in her time of Matrescence (the process of becoming a mother in mind and body) and really in the first year as you both find your feet. It can be useful to bring some awareness into the equation where well-meaning relatives are concerned.

It's never easy expressing to a parent that they need to "keep their opinions to themselves for a while" but this is an ideal time to take courage and do just that.

Why not talk to your partner about this and make some notes below to keep and remind yourself of what she needs and doesn't need at this time. Sometimes, it pays to understand that a new mother may well be doing what she can to do it all and you may see her getting exhausted from it, so have a think about what you can say and do to rescue the situation if needed.

Write your thoughts here:

Priorities

It can really help to have a written list of priorities. Having them in your head just won't cut the mustard when you are tired and going into 'freeze mode'.

Go for it here:

Never a last word...

This guide is merely that, a guide. A resource for you to find your feet as you cruise through the challenges and the joys of parenthood.

Years ago, there was more of a village mentality when it came to supporting new parents, but now many have not got that. Although it was assumed that men didn't talk about their feelings, they would go to the pub after work and offload their day with their mates. This is a vital part of parenting; talking about it. So have a think about your 'village' and who you can talk to. Perhaps note them down in the box below.

A more modern substitute for a pub is an online group or app where you can share your thoughts and feelings with other parents and support each other. The Beyond Birth Mindful Parents (Private Facebook Group) connected to this guide is one place, or how about the DAD AF (https://www.dadaf.co.uk) app for some amazing resources, ideas and chat with other Dad's and Partners.

Don't forget to check the dads and partners section in the resources section!

THE MAMMA COACH

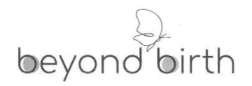

beyond birth

Helpful questionnaires

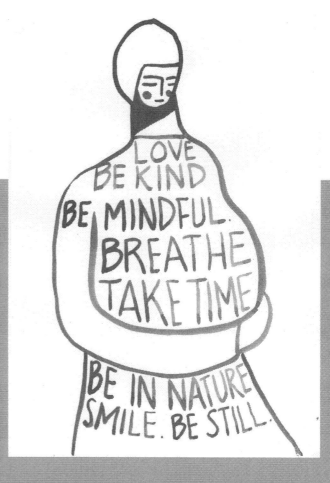

Self relationship

What does it mean to you to have a baby?

What do you need to let go of?

What do you need to do to prepare mentally?

What do you need to do to prepare physically?

What do you need to do to prepare emotionally?

Partner relationship

Here are some things to think about and perhaps discuss with your partner.

How will this baby change your relationship with your partner?

What do you need from each other to find balance? And how will you support each other?

What do you need to let go of? What's holding you back?

THE MAMMA COACH

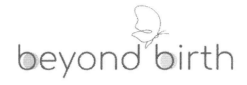

Resources

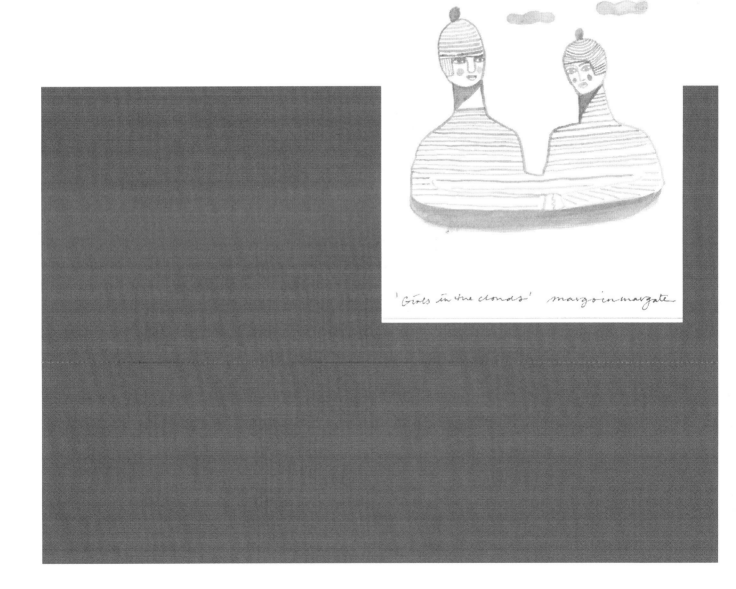

'Girls in the clouds' margo in margate

These resources are by no means an exhausted list and are currently fairly UK specific. There are so many incredible experts on the postnatal period, and I suggest you trial and error until you find what suits you individually. My recommendation is to take what you need from any advice, but always listen to your intuition and if in doubt reach out to an expert.

Beyond Birth Guide - This guide comes with 11 audios. For Exclusive access see here:
https://www.themammacoach.com/beyond-birth-guide-all-audio
Password: BeyondBirthAudio

Useful App's and Media

The Nourish App: https://www.thenourishapp.com/

Calm: https://www.calm.com/

Headspace: https://www.headspace.com/

Mindful Magazine: https://www.mindful.org/magazine/

Motherdom Magazine: https://motherdom.co.uk/

NCT: https://www.nct.org.uk/life-parent

Peppy: https://www.peppy.health/

This is Nave: thisisnave.com/

Pause, Purpose, Play Podcast by The Thomas Connection

DAD AF: www.dadaf.co.uk

The Good Enough Mother: www.drsophiebrock.com/podcast/

THE MAMMA COACH

Dads / Partners

DAD AF app: www.dadaf.co.uk

Andrew Myers: http://www.andrewmayers.info/fathers-mental-health.html

Dad's Matter: https://www.dadsmatteruk.org/

Fatherhood Institute: http://www.fatherhoodinstitute.org/

Father's Reaching Out: http://www.reachingoutpmh.co.uk/

The Hub of Hope is a database of services in the UK and NHS Mental health helplines are national organisations it is good to know so you can feel confident in having a conversation with the father: https://hubofhope.co.uk/

PMH Families: https://twitter.com/PMHfamiliesAPNI: https://apni.org/postnatal-depression-dads/

Postpartum Support International: https://www.postpartum.net/get-help/resources-for-fathers/

The Dads Net: www.thedadsnet.com

The Journal for men: https://www.mindjournals.com/products/the-journal

Beyond Birth Guide - Exclusive audio access
https://www.themammacoach.com/beyond-birth-guide-all-audio
Password: BeyondBirthAudio

THE MAMMA COACH

Support/Mental Health/ Recovery

Pandas Foundation UK: http://www.pandasfoundation.org.uk/

Anxiety & Depression Form, GAD7 and PHQ9 FORM:
https://www.efficacy.org.uk/therapy/phq-9-and-gad-7/

Make Birth Better: https://www.makebirthbetter.org/

Association for Postnatal Illness: https://apni.org/

Maternal Mental Health Alliance:
https://maternalmentalhealthalliance.org/

Maternity Action: https://maternityaction.org.uk/

Mental Health Foundation: https://www.mentalhealth.org.uk/

Mothers at home Matter: https://mothersathomematter.co.uk/

MIND: https://www.mind.org.uk/media/34727130/pnd-and-perinatal-mh-2016-pdf-version.pdf

Netmums: https://www.netmums.com/support/pre-and-postnatal-depression

NCT: https://www.nct.org.uk/life-parent

RC Psych: https://www.rcpsych.ac.uk/mental-health/problems-disorders

Unwanted intrusive thoughts: https://drcarolineboyd.com/infant-related-harm-thoughts

Dr Rebecca Moore: Perinatal Psychiatry and Birth Trauma:
https://www.doctorrebeccamoore.com/

Maternal Journal FREE guides: https://www.maternaljournal.org/

Recommended books

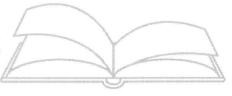

- Let's Talk About The First Year of Pregnancy, Amy Brown
- The Little Book of Self Care for New Mums, Beccy Hands & Alexis Strictland
- Why Love Matters, Sue Gerhardt
- The Self Care Revolution, Suzy Reading
- Gentle Parenting, Sarah Ockwell-Smith
- The Book You Wish Your Parents Had Read, Philippa Perry
- The Mindful Breastfeeding Book, Anna Le Grange
- Intuitive Living, Pandora Paloma
- Mindfulness for Women, Vidyamala Burch & Claire Irvin
- What No One Tells You, Aleksandra Sacks MD & Catherine Birndorf, MD
- Infant Massage, Vimala McClure
- The Fourth Trimester, Kimberly Ann Johnson
- Five Deep Breaths, The Power of Mindful Parenting, Dr Genevieve Von Lob
- The Supermum Myth, Anya Hayes and Dr Rachel Andrew
- Real Love, Sharon Salzberg
- The Baby Reflux Lady's Survival Guide, Aine Homer
- Mindfulness for Mums, Izzy Judd
- Daddy Blues, Mark Williams
- Fatherlight, Poetic Voices of Fatherhood, Blossom & Berry
- The Newborn Mother, Kate Thirlwall & Tim Smyth
- The Happiness Planner: https://thehappinessplanner.co.uk/

Infant Mental Health (parent)

Infant Foundation: https://www.mentalhealth.org.uk/

Parenthood In Mind: Specialist Perinatal Psychological Services, https://www.parenthoodinmind.co.uk/

Baby Centre - "Your Baby and the 4th Trimester": https://www.babycentre.co.uk/a25019365/your-baby-and-the-fourth-trimester

A Survival Guide to the 4th Trimester - NY Times: https://www.nytimes.com/2018/07/11/well/a-survival-guide-for-the-fourth-trimester.html

Add some of your own

Useful contacts

Please note that I have not included details of individual therapists or coaches. The websites of organisations such as the British Association for Counselling and Psychotherapy and the British Psychological Society provide the facility to search for a registered practitioner, and they also provide information on how to find a therapist. I strongly recommend that you go through these channels to find the right therapist for you.

Association for Improvements in the Maternity Service (AIMS)

AIMS is an organisation that campaigns for better birth choices. The AIMS journal is a great source of information on maternity issues.
www.aims.org.uk

Association for Post-Natal Illness (APNI)

APNI is a registered charity, it provides information leaflets, both for those experiencing postnatal illness and for healthcare professionals. It has a network of volunteers who have experienced postnatal illness themselves.
www.apni.org and www.pni.org.uk

Australian Birth Trauma Association (ABTA)

This Australian charity was established in 2016 to support women and their families who are suffering postnatally from physical and/or psychological trauma resulting from the birth process. It also offers education and support for health professionals who work with pre- and postnatal women.
www.birthtrauma.org.au

Birthrights

Is the UK's only organisation dedicated to improving women's experience of pregnancy and childbirth by promoting respect for human rights.
www.birthrights.org.uk

THE MAMMA COACH

The Birth Trauma Association (BTA)

The BTA supports all women who have had a traumatic birth experience. The website contains birth stories, information on birth trauma, a reading list and details of counsellors who specialise in birth trauma.
www.birthtraumaassociation.org.uk

The British Association for Counselling and Psychotherapy (BACP)

The BACP is a professional body for counsellors and psychotherapists in the UK. You can search their database of registered therapists by area and specialist subject - read their section on 'Finding the right therapist' for information on how to find an accredited practitioner who's right for you.
www.bacp.co.uk

The British Psychological Society (BPS)

You can use its 'Find a psychologist' pages on the website to find practictitioners who specialise in PTSD or PND in your area, and also to check that they are registered.
www.bps.org.uk

EMDR Association UK & Ireland

Eye Movement Desensitisation and Reprocessing (EMDR) is a powerful therapy designed to help people recover from traumatic events in their lives. EMDR is recognised by the World Health Organisation (WHO) and the National Institute for Health and Care Excellence (NICE). You can find accredited therapists and experienced mental health professionals on their website.
www.emdrassociation.org.uk

THE MAMMA COACH

Fathers Reaching Out

Founder Mark Williams campaigns for better support for fathers' mental health,

www.reachingoutpmh.co.uk

The Lullaby Trust

The Lullaby Trust raises awareness, provides expert advice on safer sleep for babies and offers emotional support for families.

www.lullabytrust.org.uk

Mind

Mind is England's and Wales's leading mental-health charity, which exists to help anyone with any kind of mental illness, including PND.

www.mind.org.uk

The Scottish Association for Mental Health

SAMH is Scotland's leading mental-health charity, which exists to help anyone with any kind of mental illness, including PND

www.samh.org.uk

Inspire

Inspire is Northern Ireland's leading mental-health and wellbeing charity, which exists to help anyone with any kind of illness, including PND.

www.inspirewellbeing.org

THE MAMMA COACH

Mumsnet

A website used by thousands of parents with conversations covering every kind of topic you can think of. Mumsnet can be a fantastic source of support for those with birth trauma or PND and those having trouble adjusting to parenthood. However it has caused some controversy as the comments are largely unmoderated, so you may not get the answer you're looking for or end up in a debate. But generally the community is extremely supportive and welcoming. If you're feeling vulnerable it's probably a good idea to steer clear.
www.mumsnet.com

Netmums

Another board used by thousands of parents, Netmums is more heavily moderated than Mumsnet. It also has a special area where mums can arrange meet-ups.
www.netmums.com

Family Lives

This is a national charity dedicated to helping mothers and fathers in all aspects of parenting. The website has lots of useful information and advice.
www.familylives.org.uk

Prevention and Treatment of Traumatic Childbirth (PATTCh)

PATTCh is a US charity that aims to expand awareness and advance knowledge about traumatic birth and its adverse impact on babies and childbearing people.
www.pattch.org

Post Natal Illness

This information website isrun by those affected by postnatal illness abd those who have come through it, for others in the same situation.
www.oni.org.uk

THE MAMMA COACH

Relate

Relate offers advice, relationship counselling, sex therapy, workshops, meditation, consultations and support face to face, by phone and through its website.

www.relate.org.uk

Samaritans

The Smaritans provide confidential emotional support 24 hours a day (116 123) to those experiencing despair, distress or suicidal feelings. It can sometimes help to write down your thoughts and feelings, you can email jo@samaritans.org

www.samaritans.com

Trauma and Birth Stress (TABS)

This New Zealand based organisation has a wealth of information about PTSD, including up-to-date research and parents' stories. It's also a point of contact for professionals wishing to find people who might be willing to share their experiences for research purposes.

www.tabs.org.nz

Twins and Multiple Births Association (TAMBA)

This is a great resource for parents of twins or more, providing information and suport networks.

www.tamba.org.uk

Here for you.

I hope you've found this guidebook useful. Thank you for letting me guide you on your personal journey.

Please know that you are loved and there is always someone out there who cares, however it can feel.

Reach out. There is no weakness in asking someone to listen to you, only strength in asking and pushing through any stigma around yours or other peoples ideas of mental health.

The Resources section has plenty of ideas for you, and I offer online coaching and therapy sessions. Do add your own local and national resources into the book for your reference too. There's no shame in reaching out. It's a strength, not a weakness.

Personally, I have therapy and coaching sessions monthly just as I do a yoga class for my physical health. I consider it part of taking care of myself on every level, that is not to say you need to do the same at all, it's merely some of my ways to keep my mental wellbeing in check.

Peace and smiles to you from me. Get in touch if you need to.
Take care of you.

🌐 themammacoach.com

📷 themammacoach

f themammacoach

Acknowledgements

I have so many people to thank for their support in the creation of Beyond Birth, the guide, the groups and the practitioner training.

I have to start with my boys and PB, who have been my support, inspiration and who have seen me through the tough times and brought so many loving-joyous moments that have kept me going with the crazy flow of life as a parent and entrepreneur.

Katie Carr, who has been a firm support as my VA, design whizz and business visionary. Katie's belief in me and my abilities has carved this out from the many notes and ideas to becoming a reality.

Gayle Berry, my business coach, who as such a kindred, gave me hope and helped me to see the possibilities.

Suzy Ashworth for giving me the confidence to carve out my message and see my mission clearly, and Anna le Grange for being a friend, colleague and inspiration to keep going and trust in my passion.

To my professional pals for their support and belief in me, my why and my mission: Dr Sophie Brock aka The Good Enough Mother, Mark Williams, Fathers Reaching Out and Dr Jane Hanley, Perinatal Mental Health Training, for their support and sharing their ecourse.

Sara Johnson, Connect to Calm for her amazing Yoga Nidra, Sara Campin, for including me on her team at The Nourish App and constantly sharing me words.

More acknowledgements

Dr Rebecca Moore for her review and support, Dr Caroline Boyd for her kind words and her work around Intrusive Thoughts in the perinatal period.

Liz Stanford, The Calm Birth School for her belief and support in Beyond Birth and it's ethos.

Kate Thirlwall for sharing her beautiful poems in the Beyond Birth Guide.

Victoria Jane Kearney for her beautiful and inspiring music on the Beyond Birth Guide.

Laura, Sam and Team at Maternal Journal.

Karen McMillan for her inspiring poetry in the Beyond Birth Guide.

To Margo McDaid (aka @margoinmargate) for her generous donation of the beautiful illustrations included in this guide - and her honest belief in me and my mission.

Lastly, to all those who have allowed me to hold space for them, who have reached out to me and all the kindreds who have joined the Beyond Birth Collective to come together and shout from the rooftops that parental mental wellbeing matters and we can simply and effectively change ours and other parents lives by making small, feel-good steps to find our flow in life as parents - and our children will be so much more mentally resilient and connected as a result. And to you. For being here now. Supporting yourself by working through this guide. Thank you. x.

Printed in Great Britain
by Amazon

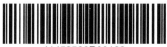

41458522R00128